Basic methods for assessment of renal fluoride excretion in community prevention programmes for oral health

2014

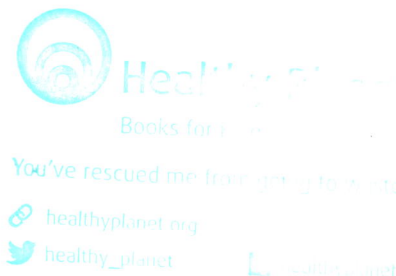
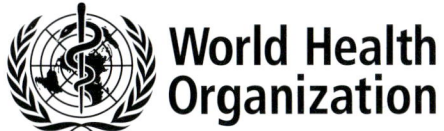
World Health
Organization

WHO Library Cataloguing-in-Publication Data

Basic methods for assessment of renal fluoride excretion in community prevention programmes for oral health.

1. Fluoride – adverse effects. 2. Fluoride – metabolism. 3. Fluoridation. 4. Fluorosis, Dental – prevention and control. 5. Community Dentistry. 6. Oral Health. 7. Program Evaluation – methods. I. World Health Organization.

ISBN 978 92 4 154870 0   (NLM classification: WU 270)

PRINTED IN FRANCE

Contents

Tables

Figures

Acronyms and abbreviations

bw	body weight
CV	coefficient of variation
CDTA	1,2-cyclohexylenedinitrilotetraacetic acid
DUFE	daily urinary fluoride excretion
F	fluoride
F.W.	formula weight
HPLC	high-performance liquid chromatography
ID	identification
IRB	institutional review boards
PABA	para-amino benzoic acid
ppm	parts per million
SD	standard deviation
TISAB	total ionic strength adjusting buffer
WHA	World Health Assembly
WHO	World Health Organization

Preface

Dental caries is still a major oral health problem in most industrialized countries, affecting 60–90% of schoolchildren and the vast majority of adults. It is also the most prevalent oral disease in several Asian and Latin American countries, although it appears to be less common and less severe in most African countries. In light of changing living conditions, however, it is expected that the incidence of dental caries will increase in many developing countries in Africa, particularly as a result of a growing consumption of sugars and inadequate exposure to fluorides. The World Health Organization (WHO) *World oral health report 2003* (*1*) noted that dental caries can be controlled by the joint action of communities, professionals and individuals aimed at reducing the impact of sugar consumption and emphasizing the beneficial effect of fluorides. In many developing countries, access to oral health services is limited; likewise, in developed countries, significant numbers of population groups are underserved.

The effects of fluoride on oral health have been studied for about a century, and the scientific literature shows that fluoride may have both beneficial and detrimental effects. The WHO policy on fluoride is clarified in various scientific articles (*2*), technical reports (*3*) and World Health Assembly resolutions (*4–6*). In 2007, for the first time in 25 years, oral health was subject to discussion by the World Health Assembly and the Executive Board of WHO (*7*). At the 60th World Health Assembly, Member States agreed on an action plan for oral health – *Oral health: Action plan for promotion and integrated disease prevention* (*8*). The resolution calls upon countries that do not have access to optimal levels of fluoride, and have not yet established fluoridation programmes, to consider the development and implementation of such programmes, giving priority to equitable strategies through automatic administration of fluoride (i.e. in drinking water, salt or milk), and to the provision of affordable fluoride toothpaste. Use of water fluoridation for prevention of dental caries began in the 1940s in USA; it has been the source of numerous studies, and has expanded to several countries around the world (*2*). Use of salt fluoridation for dental caries prevention began in Switzerland in the mid-1950s, and has been adopted by several countries around the globe (*9*). Salt fluoridation has been as effective as water fluoridation in reducing dental caries in areas where salt production and distribution can be controlled. Milk fluoridation has also proven successful in dental caries prevention, particularly in school-age children living in areas where the fluoride concentration in drinking water is suboptimal (*10*).

Population-wide automatic fluoridation measures are effective and are the most equitable ways to prevent dental caries. However, some degree of unsightly enamel fluorosis results when children are exposed to fluoride above optimal concentrations. Several products or elements containing fluoride can be sources of exposure. It is therefore important that fluoride exposure be known and health authorities be made aware of exposure before the introduction of any fluoridation or supplementation programmes for prevention of dental caries (*11*).

Total fluoride exposure of individuals or populations can be monitored by assessing fluoride concentration in plasma, urine or ductal saliva. The amount of fluoride in these biological liquids is indicative of the level of total fluoride exposure. After intake of fluoride – whether through drinking water, dietary components or fluoride supplements – the plasma fluoride level will rise immediately, but it starts to decrease within 30–60 minutes, and reverts to the original level within 3–6 hours.

Urinary fluoride excretion is basically dependent on the fluoride concentrations or rather on the concentration peaks in the plasma. In the case of long-lasting collections (e.g. 6–10 hours), the peaks tend to level out and the variations in the accumulated urine are smaller. The main advantage of using urinary fluoride excretion to estimate total fluoride exposure is that urine collections are non-invasive – no blood needs to be taken – and are thus more suitable than other methods for monitoring community fluoridation schemes. Unique field experience has been gained by using fluoride excretion in urine to evaluate programmes implementing water, salt and milk fluoridation (*11*). It is possible to develop excretion thresholds; that is, levels that should not be exceeded if unsightly enamel fluorosis is to be avoided. In programmes where fluoride is added to milk and to salt, urinary studies will identify instances of insufficient excretion, indicating suboptimal fluoride levels. Most importantly, studies of urinary fluoride provide a simple and reliable means of ensuring that total fluoride intake from all sources does not exceed certain limits; this is especially critical in young children whose permanent anterior teeth are developing (*11*).

In 1999, the WHO Oral Health Programme published the booklet *Monitoring of renal fluoride excretion in community prevention programmes in oral health* (*11*). The manual has been useful as a guide for monitoring fluoride excretion and concentrations in programmes in which either salt or milk has been used as a vehicle for administering fluoride for caries prevention. This current manual – entitled *Basic methods for assessment renal fluoride excretion in community prevention programmes for oral health* – is an update of the 1999 publication. It includes practical experience from national fluoridation programmes, and will primarily be useful in helping countries to plan effective surveillance of fluoride exposure. It is hoped that the manual will stimulate oral health personnel and public health administrators to use a systematic approach to managing and analysing data obtained from different levels of fluoride exposure. It is also a hope that the manual will motivate inter-country collaboration on efforts to establish standardized and effective epidemiological surveillance systems for community prevention programmes using fluoride. The present manual thereby complements the WHO "Oral Health Surveys – Basic Methods" (*12*), which provide recommendations on oral health assessment of population groups and specify the tools important to surveillance of oral health.

Acknowledgements

This manual was prepared by Dr R.J. Baez, University of Texas, Health Science Center, San Antonio Dental School, Texas, United States of America; Dr P.E. Petersen, WHO, Geneva, Switzerland; and Dr T.M. Marthaler, University of Zurich, Zurich, Switzerland.

Special thanks for technical advice are due to Dr V. Zohoori, Health and Social Care Institute, Teesside University, Middlesbrough, United Kingdom of Great Britain and Ireland (UK); Dr A. Rugg-Gunn, Dental School, Newcastle University, Newcastle, UK; Dr M. Buzalaf, Dental School, University of Sao Paulo, Sao Paulo, Brazil; Dr A. Villa, Institute of Nutrition, Santiago, Chile; Dr T.D. Hai, National Institute of Odontostomatology, Hanoi, Viet Nam; and Dr P. Phanthumvanit, Thammasat University, Faculty of Dentistry, Pathumtani, Thailand.

Financial support

This report was published with the financial support from the Borrow Foundation, United Kingdom. The World Health Organization Oral Health Programme, Geneva, is grateful for the continued support to activities for global oral health.

1 Introduction

1.1 Background

Fluoride is a natural constituent of all types of human diet and is present, in varying amounts, in drinking water throughout the world. Because of its value in preventing decay (i.e. formation of dental caries), fluoride is increasingly being used for this purpose in several countries. Enamel fluorosis (unsightly mottling of the teeth) is the only untoward effect of the use of fluoride, and the condition is known to occur in regions worldwide wherever drinking water contains high levels of fluoride naturally.

Most of the time throughout the day, teeth are bathed in saliva; hence, the teeth benefit from fluoride ions present in the oral environment, originating from a number of sources to which the individual may be exposed. The concentration of fluoride in saliva varies among individuals, and depends on various factors such as salivary secretion rate and the type of fluoride exposure. To exert a cariostatic effect, fluoride levels need to rise above the predominantly low level several times throughout the day. When fluoride is added to vehicles such as water, salt or milk, it becomes available in the oral cavity at optimal levels several times a day, whereas toothbrushing with fluoride-containing toothpaste provide concentrated fluoride twice a day. These methods of fluoride supplementation are highly successful in reducing levels of dental caries in entire populations. Fluoride is also available through concentrated gels, rinsing solutions, lacquers or varnishes. These methods are most appropriate for selective use on individuals who are suffering from high caries activity.

The goals of community-based public health programmes should be to implement measures that raise the fluoride concentration in as many mouths as possible as often as possible, using the most appropriate method. Effective methods are water, salt or milk fluoridation either alone or in combination with fluoride-containing toothpaste, all of which make fluoride available to the population in a manner that does not require cooperative effort or direct action. However, when fluoride is ingested by young children, very mild dental enamel fluorosis may occur. Because of the numerous sources of fluoride available today, the risk of enamel fluorosis must always be borne in mind. Thus, public health administrators should assess the total fluoride exposure of the population before introducing any additional fluoridation or supplementation programmes for caries prevention.

The overall goals of this document are to provide information on:

- determining current levels of fluoride exposure;
- determining the appropriateness of fluoride-based caries-prevention programmes;
- using fluoride in urine as a biomarker of fluoride exposure; and
- assessing adherence to fluoride-based community preventive programmes.

Specific objectives are to:

- present the concept of urinary fluoride as a biomarker of fluoride exposure;
- provide guidance on the general design of urinary fluoride assessment, including identification of participants, sampling, methods of monitoring, methods of time-controlled urine collection (24-hoururine collection and timed collections of urine obtained from defined periods of a day) and number of subjects suggested;
- describe the methods for urinary collection, and the elements needed for both sample collection and the determination of fluoride in urine (and in water, if required);
- provide advice on data management and evaluation of results using simple calculations;
- provide an option for countries that have a special interest in conducting a more comprehensive analysis of data;
- provide information and examples of recording other sources of fluoride exposure, if such is indicated by any specific situation; and
- provide guidance on design of the final report.

1.2 Sources of fluoride intake in humans

Years ago, water was the main source of fluoride exposure to humans, although other sources of fluoride were recognized, including the environment and pollution from industrial emissions. Today, there are many sources of fluoride, and this needs to be taken into consideration when planning a community caries prevention programme using fluoride. Fluoride-containing toothpaste can be a significant source of fluoride ingestion, particularly in young children who involuntarily or voluntarily swallow considerable portions of the toothpaste, either because the swallowing reflex in young children is not fully developed, or because some toothpastes are formulated to heave candy-like flavours (*3, 13*).

1.3 Fluoride metabolism and excretion

The fluoride content of the human body is determined by certain physiological relationships. Urinary fluoride concentration and excretion depend on plasma fluoride levels; they are also influenced by urinary flow and pH. The rate of fluoride excretion depends on the amount of bioavailable fluoride ingested; that is, the fluoride actually absorbed by the organism and distributed in the bloodstream. Urinary pH is affected by diet. For example, diets high in vegetables lead to more alkaline urine, resulting in a higher proportion of ingested fluoride being excreted in urine. Conversely, diets rich in meat lead to more acid urine, resulting in a lower proportion of ingested fluoride being excreted in urine. In spite of these confounding factors, determination of renal fluoride excretion in young children is a useful method for estimating total fluoride exposure in community programmes for caries prevention that use water, milk or salt fluoridation.

From data obtained in studies of ingested (systemic) fluoride – mainly via water, milk or salt – it is possible to develop excretion thresholds; that is, levels that should not be exceeded (Section 5.6, Table 5.3). Urinary studies will also identify instances of insufficient excretion, indicating suboptimal fluoride levels. However, most importantly, studies of urinary fluoride provide a simple means of ensuring that the total fluoride intake from all sources does not exceed certain limits, especially in young children whose permanent teeth are developing. This is essential in order to avoid unsightly dental enamel fluorosis.

1.4 Biomarkers of fluoride exposure

Recent reviews have considered the suitability of biomarkers for fluoride exposure. One review looked at contemporary biomarkers (i.e. those measuring present or very recent exposure) (*14*), and looked at biomarkers for both recent and historical exposure (*15, 16*). The contemporary biomarkers considered were blood, bone surface, saliva, milk, sweat and urine; the biomarkers of recent exposure considered were nails and hair; and the biomarkers of historical exposure considered were bone and teeth. The reviews concluded that, at present, urine is the most useful biomarker of contemporary fluoride exposure. The recent review on contemporary biological markers of exposure to fluoride stated:

A proportion of ingested fluoride is excreted in urine. Plots of daily urinary fluoride excretion against total daily fluoride intake suggest that daily urinary fluoride excretion is suitable for predicting fluoride intake for groups of people, but not individuals. While fluoride concentrations in plasma, saliva and urine have some ability to predict fluoride exposure, present data are insufficient to recommend utilizing fluoride concentrations in these body fluids as biomarkers of contemporary fluoride exposure for individuals. Daily fluoride excretion in urine can be considered a useful biomarker of contemporary fluoride exposure for groups of people, and normal values have been published (*14*).

Thus, the value of urinary fluoride as a biomarker of fluoride exposure has been established and its limitations have been documented.

1.5 Urinary fluoride assessments in population oral health

Ingested fluoride from all sources, whether deliberately or unintentionally ingested, is excreted primarily in the urine. Thus, studies of urinary fluoride levels are ideal for assessing the intake of fluoride in populations. More particularly, such studies also provide a basis for decisions on the use of fluoride for caries prevention.

The mechanisms of the absorption of fluoride are well known. When fluoride is ingested via water, in a tablet (or supplement) or in fluoride-containing toothpaste on an empty stomach, the fluoride concentration in the blood reaches a peak after about 30 minutes, and returns to the usual level after 90–180 minutes. If fluoride is ingested with rice cooked with fluoridated salt in the course of a main meal, the peak is likely to occur after one hour, and it may take 3–4 hours for the fluoride to return to the usual level. Taking into account these and similar variations throughout the day, it is evident that 24-hour collections of urine are the best basis for estimating fluoride exposure. Thus, whenever it can be organized in a given situation, 24-hour urine should be collected.

Recently, the relationship between fluoride excretion and fluoride intake was investigated systematically in relatively large numbers of children and adults (*17*). The study examined all published data pairs of total daily fluoride intake and the corresponding daily urinary fluoride excretion from 212 children aged less than 7 years and 283 adults aged 18–75 years. Analyses of these data indicated that an average of 45% of ingested fluoride was excreted in urine in children; for adults, the corresponding figure was 74%. These data provide the means for converting 24-hour fluoride intake into 24-hour urinary fluoride excretion (*14*). Fluoride intakes of between 0.05 and 0.07 mg/kg body weight (bw)/day are accepted as "optimal", whereas intakes above 0.1 mg/kg bw/day increase the risk of enamel fluorosis (*18*).

9

Table 5.3 (Section 5.6) shows the lower and upper margins of optimal intake according to Villa's equation for selected age groups of children (*17*). According to the equation, for fluoride levels to be optimal, children in the age group 3–5 years (normally having a weight of 17.3 kg) should have an average daily fluoride excretion of 0.33–0.45 mg/day. Table 5.4 shows the calculated daily urinary fluoride excretion (DUFE) associated with low, optimal and high fluoride intake for ages 1–14 years for each year of age, and Table 5.5 presents the calculated DUFE associated with low, optimal and high fluoride intake for broader age groups.

1.6   Areas of uncertainty

Several areas of uncertainty are associated with the use of urinary fluoride as a biomarker of fluoride exposure. These uncertainties, listed below, should be considered when planning, conducting and interpreting the findings of studies of urinary fluoride excretion.

- *Influence of diet on urinary fluoride excretion.* As discussed in Section 1.3, communities consuming diets high in vegetables are likely to excrete urine that is more alkaline than urine excreted by those consuming a diet high in meats. Higher alkalinity results in excretion of a higher proportion of ingested fluoride. Thus, in communities with a high vegetable intake, a relatively high fluoride excretion does not necessarily imply a high fluoride intake.
- *Within-subject variation.* It is usual to collect urine from subjects for 1 day only; hence, there will be considerable within-subject variation in the results; and this within-subject variation can be as large as between-subject variation. Thus, within-subject variation can inflate the range and variance of data from urine excretion studies. To limit such effects, it would be necessary to record results over several days for each subject. In practice, this is rarely necessary because there is little effect on the mean values, but it does imply that ranges and variances need to be interpreted cautiously. Reports must note the potential effects of within-subject variation, to avoid misinterpretation of data presented as ranges of fluoride excretion and intakes.
- *Lack of correlation between urinary fluoride excretion and fluoride intake.* Urinary fluoride excretion is **not** suitable for predicting fluoride intake for individuals (see Section 1.4: "Biomarkers of fluoride intake").
- *Uncertainty about levels needed to provide protection.* The so-called "optimal" fluoride intake recommended for children has an empirical origin; nevertheless, the actual range that is sufficient to protect against caries and beyond which dental enamel fluorosis may happen is not known precisely.

● *Methodological errors.* If the method chosen is a timed period collection of urine covering 8–18 hours of the 24-hour cycle, an error will be associated with the estimation of 24-hour fluoride excretion in urine from such data.

2   General design of study

2.1   Background

The rate of urinary excretion of fluoride varies throughout the day and night, depending on the time of fluoride ingestion, particularly where fluoride-containing toothpaste is used and is perhaps swallowed during brushing, and where a fluoride supplement is given once a day (e.g. in the form of tablets or fluoridated milk). Therefore, when using urine to evaluate fluoride excretion, it is best to collect the urine for the entire 24-hour period. Shorter periods can be used if necessary, but the limitations of this approach must be recognized (see Section 1.6). There may be special circumstances where information on pH of urine is useful (see Sections 1.3 and 1.6), but certain safeguards are required in order to obtain a valid estimate of pH in fresh urine, as discussed in Sections 3.2.1 and 4.1.

2.2   Identification of participants

Countries contemplating the introduction of additional fluoridation or supplementation programmes should consider measurement of urinary excretion as an important element of studies of total fluoride exposure. Such studies should include identification of community water supplies and mapping of their fluoride concentration, use of fluoride supplements, use and frequency of fluoride-containing toothpastes, and identification of any other possible sources of fluoride to which the target population may be exposed.

2.3   Sampling

A study of fluoride excretion may be undertaken for various purposes such as community surveillance, field demonstration trial or research. The selection of individuals to participate in each type of investigation will depend on the specific purpose, and both the purpose and the basis of selection should be clearly established before the study begins. If the study is for community surveillance, the population should be selected randomly, because elements of the diet that affect fluoride intake (e.g. water, salt and dietary habits) may vary with area and with socioeconomic status. Where total randomization is impossible, a careful selection of subjects must be made from multiple sites, taking into account any special or predominant regional dietary habits.

Sampling procedures should consider location, number of subjects, age group, frequency, and time of study and number of days; these criteria are discussed below.

Location

The study population should be representative of the community in terms of fluoride exposure and dietary habits. It may be useful to target certain population groups living in different sections of the community that have different behavioural or environmental conditions.

Number of subjects

The total number of participants will depend on the scale of programme or type of investigation. For the 24-hour urine collection method, a general recommendation is to recruit 30–50 subjects at each location or site. If for example 10 important sites are identified in the community 300–500 individuals may be needed for the sample. This number may be relevant for 24-hour urinary fluoride excretion in the population of a given age; however, numbers outside this range may be appropriate, depending on the scale of programme or type of community study. It may be preferable to establish a sample for children and a sample for adults, thus in that case up to 600–1000 individuals are needed. However, surveys based on a high number of individuals may be time consuming and less practical to carry out in community programmes. Therefore, even larger samples call for shorter urine collection periods, for example, 8 hours or 14–16 hours.

In all urinary excretion studies care should be taken to minimize drop-outs and incomplete data. The figure of 30–50 subjects per site is based on the fact that renal fluoride excretion is dominated by simple physical and chemical rules, and that "biological" variations are subordinate (disturbances of fluoride excretion are rare, particularly in the first two decades of life). In the hundreds of studies that have been conducted, excretion was primarily dependent on the fluoride intake. Almost no cases had unexpected results, and the amount of fluoride excreted (or, in older studies, the urinary fluoride concentration) was always in the expected range. Cases of outliers with very high fluoride excretions were only reported where a child had swallowed large numbers of fluoride lozenges or several grams of fluoride-containing dentifrice.

As noted in Section 2.2, a country may have several factors that may influence fluoride intake, such as special dietary habits, socioeconomic status, and environmental conditions; because these factors may be unknown, the study population should be selected at random. Where the conditions are known (e.g. in regions with high fluoride concentration in the water), a careful selection of the study population must be made from multiple sites.

Age groups

If the study is conducted to assist on planning effective surveillance of fluoride exposure in fluoridation programmes priority is given to children of the younger ages because of their susceptibility to enamel fluorosis. The following groups require special attention:

- toilet-trained children who can provide urine collections up to the age of 6 years, or even 4 years, because this would include children at ages when the susceptibility to dental enamel fluorosis is greatest;
- non-toilet-trained children, that is, those in nappies (diapers);
- children aged over 6 years.
- adults, exposed to fluoride in certain industries (for instance aluminium production, addition of fluoride to water, salt or milk, or exposed to drinking water with excessively high fluoride concentrations).

Frequency

Urinary fluoride excretion studies on the target population should be conducted before and after the start of the fluoridation programme. Fluoride excretion begins to rise immediately after the start of a fluoride programme, but takes a few weeks or months to reach a steady state. One reason for this is that the skeleton accumulates some of the additional fluoride intake, so it takes a few weeks for a "steady state" to be reached. Thus, for milk fluoridation programmes, evaluation 1 month after the start of the programme may be appropriate. However, for water fluoridation programmes it may be advisable to wait longer, to allow fluoridated water to work its way through the water supply system. In the case of salt fluoridation, it may take several months (e.g. 9 months) until non-fluoridated salt has disappeared from the shelves and is used up in the household.

Time of study and number of days

Extremes of seasonal weather conditions should be avoided. It is usual to collect urine from subjects for 1 day only, but collection over 2 days makes it possible to estimate variability both within and between subjects. Whatever the number of collection days chosen, the same number of days used be used both before and after the programme.

2.4 Methods of monitoring

The data that should be collected in urinary fluoride studies include number of subjects participating, number of successful collections, duration of collection, fluoride concentration, urinary flow and fluoride excretion; these data can be summarized in tabular format (see Table 5.1, Section 5.6). From studies of urinary fluoride conducted in several countries over recent decades, four methods of study have generally emerged as useful: 24-hour collection, 14–16-hour collection, 8-hour collection and spot sample. The 24-hour urine collection should be used wherever possible (Sections 4 and 5), but 14–16 or even 8-hour collection can be used if necessary (Sections 6 and 7). Where 24-hour or continuous supervised collection periods are not possible, spot samples of urine can sometimes provide valuable information (Section 8).

Section 2.4.1 discusses collection over 24 hours and Section 2.4.2 discusses collection over shorter time periods.

2.4.1 24-hour urine collection

The question of whether urinary fluoride excretion in a given population is at the desired level can be answered by straightforward evaluation of 24-hour urine collections. Although the calculations are simple, it is advisable to record all factors that may affect individual and group outcomes. Calculating the amount of fluoride excreted over 24 hours per subject provides an estimate of fluoride intake for groups of people; this finding can then be compared with recommended levels of fluoride intake for populations (see Section 1.5) (*14, 17*).

Usually, only one 24-hour collection is obtained per subject; however, if additional collections are taken, the results can be used to estimate within-subject variation (see Section 1.6). A 24-hour collection is usually from morning to morning, with the first void on the first morning being excluded, and the first void on the second morning being included. There are several reports describing collection of urine over 24 hours [e.g. (*19–22*)]. Complete 24-hour urine samples can be obtained through good organization and close supervision at school and at home. Several studies have reported urinary fluoride excretion in children [e.g. (*19, 21–35*)] and adults [e.g. (*36–40*)], based on 24-hour urine collection.

It is important to check the completeness of the collected 24-hour urine samples, because participants – both children and adults – may occasionally pass urine during the collection period but forget to collect it. This is one of the main sources of error, and it results in underestimation of fluoride excretion. However, efforts to seek out subjects who are "dependable" in this respect may introduce bias, meaning that the final study group may not be representative of the population.

There are three methods for checking the completeness of 24-hour collections: urine volume or flow rate, creatinine and para-amino benzoic acid (PABA). Each of these is discussed below. Because each criterion has limitations, it is best to consider more than one criterion before excluding a collection.

Urine volume or flow rate

Urine volume (or flow rate) is a commonly used marker for validating the completeness of 24-hour urine samples. For example, in children aged 2–4 years, a 24-hour urine volume of less than 140 mL or a flow rate of less than 5 mL/hour may indicate incomplete collection. However, daily urine volume, and consequently flow rate, is affected by the amount of liquid consumed per day. The upper section of Table 5.2 provides criteria that can be used in cleaning data for children aged 2–6 years.

Creatinine

Creatinine is spontaneously formed by the breakdown of creatine in muscle, and levels are only slightly affected by diet or normal physical activity. It is excreted in urine at a relatively constant rate, through glomerular filtration. In any individual with stable renal function, the scatter of serum creatinine concentrations from day to day is small, having a within-subject coefficient of variation (CV) of about 4%. Therefore, 24-hour urinary excretion of creatinine has been used as a marker of completeness of 24-hour urine collection. Samples with a 24-hour urine creatinine of less than 8 mg/kg bw/day may be due to incomplete collection, and samples with a 24-hour urine creatinine of more than 22 mg/kg bw/day may be due to collection for longer than 24 hours (see the middle section of Table 5.2).

Para-amino benzoic acid

PABA is part of the vitamin B folic acid, and is eaten in small amounts in foods such as yeast, cereals, meat and milk. Larger amounts are included in some vitamin tablets, hair dyes or sunscreens. Since PABA is fully absorbed and fully excreted in urine within 24 hours, it has been used in some large surveys, such as the United Kingdom of Great Britain and Ireland (UK) National Diet and Nutrition Survey (NDNS), to assess the completeness of 24-hour urine collection. Before administering PABA tablets, the eligibility of participants should be checked. PABA tablets should not be given to those who are pregnant; have allergy to hair dye, sunscreen or vitamins; or are taking sulphonamides. PABA may interfere with the antibacterial action of sulphonamides.

16

This method of determining completeness of the 24-hour urine sample involves providing three 80 mg PABA tablets to the participants, to be taken at specified intervals with meals. Completeness is then assessed by measuring urinary recovery of PABA over 24 hours. Collections having PABA recovery of 85–110% are considered complete (see the lower section of Table 5.2). PABA can be estimated using a colorimetric method (*41*) or a high-performance liquid chromatography (HPLC) method (*42*). The latter is preferable because some common drugs (e.g. paracetamol) cross-react in the colorimetric method, giving falsely high recoveries.

2.4.2   *Timed collections of urine obtained from defined periods of a day*

In all studies that are not based on 24-hour urine collection, information on the timing of maximum fluoride ingestion is important. Fluoride supplementation other than through drinking water usually results in peaks of fluoride excretion at certain hours. After ingestion of fluoridated milk, food containing fluoridated salt, or fluoride tablets, maximum fluoride excretion levels are generally reached within 30–180 minutes; the same is true where toothpaste is swallowed during brushing of the teeth. Information on eating habits allows for better planning of any study and facilitates the interpretation of results.

The primary purpose of the time-controlled method is to provide fairly precise estimations of 24-hour fluoride excretion when 24-hour collections are not feasible. The estimations are fairly reliable when urine collection starts during or immediately after intake of fluoridated milk or supplements. For monitoring the effects of salt fluoridation, urine collection must start shortly after consumption of the main salted meal, and collection should last at least 2 hours (3 hours if possible). By organizing an additional collection for the night, it is possible to readily obtain urine collections lasting 9–12 hours. In many such studies, a third collection during the daytime is organized for another 3–5 hours. In this way, the total duration of collections covered is between 14 hours (i.e. 2+9+3) and 20 hours (i.e. 3+12+5). The many physiological studies on plasma fluoride indicate that very high or very low fluoride excretion are not to be expected in the 4 hours (i.e. 24 minus 20) to 10 hours (i.e. 24 minus 14) for which data are not collected.

During the past 30 years, several fluoride studies based on 8-hour or 14–16-hour urine collections have been reported. The results indicate that such studies are useful for evaluating public health programmes (*20, 43–52*).

For particular purposes – such as to establish the time of day at which fluoride elimination is highest in the population of interest – it may be useful to collect urine separately for specific periods (e.g. morning, afternoon, night) and to analyse each micturition separately. In such cases, collection must include 2–3 hours that cover the period of the day when the customary main fluoride ingestion and subsequent excretion takes place.

12–20 hour collections

Collections of urine over intervals of between 12 and 20 hours should cover, as far as possible, three distinct periods in all subjects:

- **High**: a supervised sample collected during the period when maximum excretion is expected. If supplementary fluoride is given (e.g. in fluoridated milk, tablets or drops, or a meal containing fluoridated salt), collection should start as soon as possible (but at least within 30 minutes of the beginning of the meal), and should last at least 2 hours, to ensure that the excretion peak is captured.
- **Low**: a supervised sample taken during a part of the day that is not preceded by high fluoride intake.
- **Nocturnal**: a sample taken during the night (i.e. during the period of sleep). Children or their parents should bring this sample to school the next morning.

Ideally, a complete series of three collections should be collected from each subject [e.g. see (47)]. Average fluoride excretion levels should generally be similar in the **low** and **nocturnal** collections. If they differ widely, efforts should be made to determine the possible reason (e.g. young children may swallow considerable amounts of fluoride-containing toothpaste). In some developing countries, half of the children in a community go to school in the morning (from 07:00 to 11:00) and half in the afternoon (from 12:00 to 17:00). Therefore, it is likely that the first groups will provide morning and nocturnal urine samples, and the second groups afternoon and nocturnal samples. In such circumstances, acceptance of these "incomplete series" of collections may be the only way to obtain data.

8-hour collections

When it is difficult to obtain three collections covering a total of 12–20 hours, two collections extending over as many hours as possible should be the aim. Urine may be collected at school or at work, preferably under supervision, with a total duration of at least 8 hours. Two different collections are necessary, one following the main intake of fluoride (high) and one at another time (low or, preferably, nocturnal). This may be the only possibility for studies undertaken in subjects from poor areas or large cities, or from rural areas of some developing countries where it may be difficult to secure cooperation of the population. Nocturnal collections are preferable, because high nocturnal fluoride excretion is usually indicative of high 24-hour excretion, and thus of high fluoride intake.

Specific situation of young children in day care

In some countries, young children are taken to a day-care centre or pre-kinder institution in the early morning, and remain there until late morning or early afternoon; they are then transferred to the home of a relative or to a babysitter until late afternoon, when they are taken home by their parents. In these circumstances, supervised urine collection may only be possible during the morning and nocturnal periods totalling 14–15 hours. In such cases, a cautious approach is to look separately at the results during the low and high excretion periods (*43*).

3 Methods for collecting urine, and for handling and evaluating results

3.1 Recording of information

For specific studies investigating sources of fluoride exposure, it is useful to obtain and comprehensively record information on fluoride exposure, both general (i.e. factors that bear on the entire group, community or region) and personal (i.e. factors such as fluoride exposure at home or professionally applied fluorides). Less comprehensive data will suffice when evaluating the level of fluoride exposure in communities before or after the introduction of fluoride-based preventive programmes. The following subclauses provide details of relevant information to be recorded. Figures 3.1 through 3.5 depict examples that can be useful to the investigator on recruiting efforts (Figure 3.4), designing labels for urine collecting periods (Figures 3.1 and 3.2), summarizing data (Figure 3.3) and collecting information on tooth brushing practices and use of fluoride supplements (Figure 3.5).

3.1.1 General information

The fluoride content of the drinking water in the community must be ascertained. A good practice is to provide parents or guardians with a clean 25 mL plastic cylinder – labelled with the identification (ID) code assigned to the child – with a screw cap, to obtain a sample of water that the child drinks at home. Parents should be instructed to rinse the cylinder a couple of times with the water the child usually drinks at home, fill it to the top with that water, ensure that the cylinder is tightly closed, and bring the sample to the school for testing.

If milk fluoridation is present, the quantity of fluoride in milk and the time of ingestion should be established. If salt fluoridation programmes have been implemented in the country, or if fluoridated salt is otherwise available, it is essential to determine whether fluoride is added to domestic salt only, or also to the salt used in bakeries, large kitchens (e.g. in restaurants, workplace, canteens and hospitals) or the food industry (53).

Data on actual fluoride concentration in salt are also crucial. A level of 250 mg/kg is commonly used when addition of fluoride is limited to domestic

Name				Sex[a]	ID No.	
School/ institution or place of employment				Date		
Period A[b]	Time initial voiding[c]	Time	Time	Time	Time	Final time
Micturition		1	2	3	4	
Volume (mL)	▉	1	2	3	4	Volume (mL)

ID, identification

Note: In some countries it is not permitted to record the name of the child; in such cases ,the project director should maintain a cross-reference list, and the ID number assigned should be used to identify data collected from individuals.

a Sex is included merely to alert staff and ensure that a wide mouth jar is provided to female children to facilitate collection.

b The period should be designated depending whether it is the morning period (A), afternoon (B), or evening (C), and the corresponding labels printed and affixed to each jar beforehand. Other period designations may be used, but the designations must be decided on before the start of the study.

c The volume of urine at initial voiding is not recorded and is not analysed for fluoride, but the time must be carefully recorded on the label and entered in the form shown in Fig. 3.3.

Figure 3.1 Example of daytime label used in time-controlled collections, to be attached to the urine collecting jar (WHO Form No. 96392, modified)

Name_____ **ID No.**_____

Overnight urine collection   Date_____

1) **Note the time** at which subject urinated before going to bed. DO NOT COLLECT THIS URINE

    _____ pm

2) If subject wishes to urinate during the night he or she should use the jar

3) When subject gets up in the morning he or she should urinate in the jar. Then close the jar and **note the time** _____ **am**

    PLEASE BRING THE JAR TO SCHOOL IN THE MORNING

Figure 3.2 Overnight urine collection label used in time-controlled collections (WHO Form No. 96393)

General information: Region _____ Country _____ Community _____
Area: Urban _____ Rural _____ Date _____   School: _____ Code:_____ Mean temperature:____°C

Children data:						Period A (High)		Period B (Low)		Period C (Nocturnal)	
No	ID	Age	Sex	Weight		Start	End	Start	End	Start	End
					Time						
					Vol.						
					Time						
					Vol.						
					Time						
					Vol.						
					Time						
					Vol.						
					Time						
					Vol.						
					Time						
					Vol.						
					Time						
					Vol.						
					Time						
					Vol.						
					Time						
					Vol.						
					Time						
					Vol.						
					Time						
					Vol.						
					Time						
					Vol.						
					Time						
					Vol.						
					Time						
					Vol.						
					Time						
					Vol.						
					Time						
					Vol.						
					Time						
					Vol.						
					Time						
					Vol.						
					Time						
					Vol.						
					Time						
					Vol.						
					Time						
					Vol.						
					Time						
					Vol.						
					Time						
					Vol.						
					Time						
					Vol.						

Figure 3.3 Summary record form of urine collection from a group of children in time-controlled collections (WHO Form No. 96391)

Preschool, kindergarten, day-care centre or
elementary school_____

Community_____ Date _____

Dear Parent:

The school has agreed to participate in a study about fluoride and children 3–5 years old. The dental health staff from
the _____ of _____ wants to study how much fluoride children have in their
urine. Fluoride is found naturally in our drinking water. People from this community are being asked to take part in this
study because fluoride helps to prevent dental cavities. What the dental health staff learns about our community will be
compared with information from other communities and will help establishing a programme to prevent cavities (caries)
in the population living in this community.

The study is simple. It involves collecting a few samples of your child's urine and a sample of your drinking water.
Plastic containers will be provided by the people in charge of the study. Please let us know whether or not you would
be interested in getting more details and possibly agreeing that your child takes part in this activity.

We kindly ask you to complete the form below (X) and send it back with your child.

You may contact the nurse's office or your child's teacher if you have questions you want answered first.

YES   I am interest   **NO**   I am not interested

Your name _____

Contact information _____:

Figure 3.4 Sample invitation (example)

salt. However, when almost all salt destined for human consumption
(including salt used in bakeries, large kitchens and the food industry) is fluoridated, concentrations of 180–200 mg/kg are commonly used. Samples of salt
and pre-salted food must be collected from food markets, restaurants, bakeries, institutions, salt-processing plants or distributors, and so on.

Whereas some countries have collected data on salt intake, others estimate
this by salt "disappearance", which is obtained indirectly by summing home
production and imports minus quantities of exported salt, or directly from
quantities of salt sold (if this can be determined). Only a portion of salt used
in households or in large kitchens is actually ingested, and that proportion
can vary widely between different cultures. Salt as sodium chloride contains
39.3% sodium, and the maximum recommended daily intake of sodium is
2.3 g, which amounts to a maximum of 5 g salt per day (*54*).

3.1.2 Personal information

Each subject must be identified with a unique (non-repeated) sequential
number. The age recorded is usually that on the last birthday, although the
exact date of birth can be included. Sex is not mandatory, but some investigators prefer to record and report gender balance (i.e. ratio of male: female).
Body weight must be determined on the day of the sample collection to the

Figure 3.5 Questionnaire on use of fluoride supplements and toothpaste

---

Ministry of Health of _____ **Dental department** _____

Use of dentifrices and fluoride supplements by children 3–5 years of age

---

Country _____ **Community** _____

Recorder _____ **Survey date** ☐☐☐☐☐☐

Day   month   year

A. General information

---

1. **Child name** _____   2. **Date of birth** ☐☐☐☐☐☐

Day   month   year

---

3. **Age in years** ☐☐   4. **Sex**   Male ☐   Female ☐

        1   2

---

5.   **Occupation of the father or responsible family member**

Manual ....☐ 1

Technical..☐ 2

Professional..☐ 3

---

6.   **Level of education of mother**

None...☐ 1

Elementary ....☐ 2

Secondary...☐ 3

College ....☐ 4

Professional..☐ 5

Figure 3.5 *Continued*

B. Use of dentifrice

		Yes	No
7.	**Does** (*child name*) **use toothbrush?**...	☐ 1	☐ 2

		Yes	No
8.	**Does** (*child name*) **use toothpaste?**...	☐ 1	☐ 2

9. **Which toothpaste does** (*child name*) **use now?** _____

10. **At what age did** (*child name*) **start to use toothpaste?** years ☐☐

11. **How many times per day does** (*child name*) **brushes with toothpaste?** ☐ times

12. **How much toothpaste does** (*child name*) **use each time?**

☐ 1   ☐ 2   ☐ 3

13. **Who places the toothpaste on the child's toothbrush?**

The child ☐ 1   The mother or other adult ☐ 2

14.	**Does the mother or another adult supervise the child during tooth brushing?**	Yes ☐ 1	No ☐ 2

15.	**Do you usually buy the same toothpaste for the adults and children in the family?**..	Yes ☐ 1	No ☐ 2

Figure 3.5 *Continued*

16. **Which is the main reason for preferring the toothpaste brand that you buy for your child?**

Cost	☐ 1
Flavour	☐ 2
Package	☐ 3
Other	☐ 4

17. **Please tell us, what is the purpose of the toothpaste?** *(Care should be taken not to influence the answer)*

To prevent dental caries	☐ 1
To give good mouth breath	☐ 2
For cleanliness	☐ 3
Other	☐ 4

18. **Has** *(child name)* **ever taken medicines with fluoride for preventing dental caries, such as drops, tablets or vitamins?**

Fluoride drops	☐ 1
Fluoride tablets	☐ 2
Vitamins with fluoride	☐ 3

19. **Is** *(child name)* **taking any of these at the present time** ....

                                           Yes   No
                                           ☐ 1   ☐ 2

*If the answer is **No**, finish the interview.*

20. **At what age did** *(child name)* **start taking these medicines?** .... years ☐☐

    1 = Drops with fluoride   2 = Fluoride tablets   3 = Vitamins with fluoride .... ☐

Figure 3.5 *Continued*

Prenatal		Postnatal-1 (year)		Postnatal-2 (years)		Postnatal-3 (years)	
Medicine	For how long[a]	Medicine	For how long[a]	Medicine	For how long[a]	Medicine	For how long[a]
☐	☐☐	☐	☐☐	☐	☐☐	☐	☐☐
☐	☐☐	☐	☐☐	☐	☐☐	☐	☐☐
☐	☐☐	☐	☐☐	☐	☐☐	☐	☐☐

Check single box and enter number of months on boxes under "how long"

a. *A period of use is considered to be 15 days or more.*

21. **Please tell us the brand that** (*child name*) **has used** *(include a list of the medicines that exist in the market)*

    Drops ………………………………………………………… ☐ 1

    Tablets ……………………………………………………… ☐ 2

    Vitamins. …………………………………………………… ☐ 3

    Do not remember …………………………………………… ☐ 4

22. **Who prescribes use of such medicines?**

    Dentist.. ☐ 1

    Physician .... ☐ 2

    Other .... ☐ 3

23. **How many times a day does** (*child name*) **take these supplements?**

    Once .... ☐ 1

    Twice... ☐ 2

    Three times.. ☐ 3

    More than three times .... ☐ 4

Figure 3.5 *Continued*

---

24. **Where do you buy these medicines?**

   Pharmacy/Drugstore .... ☐ 1

   Dentist/Physician clinic .... ☐ 2

   Other .... ☐ 3

   Specify _____

---

25. **What is the brand name of salt you buy for the family?**_____

Thank you for your answers

nearest 0.1 kg; this can be obtained easily using a portable scale (with the subject wearing light clothing) at the same time as name tags or ID numbers are given.

Investigators may collect from parents or guardians any known information on fluoride exposure of children or directly from adult participants. Information required for the investigation of sources of fluoride exposure could include use of fluoride-containing toothpaste, whether children use adult toothpaste (1500–2500 parts per million [ppm]F) or toothpaste for children with a lower fluoride content (250–500 ppm), frequency and quantity of toothpaste use, age at which child began brushing with toothpaste, whether child brushes teeth under supervision, and use of fluoride supplements (brand name, fluoride concentration and frequency of use and quantity used). Additional information may include the use of other fluoride-containing products for oral care (e.g. fluoride rinses and regular topical application by dental professionals). The fluoride concentration in these products and the frequency of their use can be recorded in a questionnaire specially designed for this purpose (see Figure 3.5), which is administered to parents or guardians either on the same day as sample collection or at a different time. If the study is conducted as part of occupational health surveillance, information pertinent to nature of products being handled, intensity of exposure in terms of hours per day, week or months and exposure protective measures available should be recorded.

In this context, it is important to differentiate clearly between "fluoride exposure" and "fluoride intake". *Exposure* is a general term indicating availability or frequent use of fluoride (or both); *intake* is more specific, referring to the ingestion of an amount of fluoride that is known approximately or may even be measured.

3.2   Essential preparatory practices

3.2.1   Pre-collection planning approaches

Informed consent

Fluoride exposure studies involving children require informed consent from the children's parents or guardians. Collaboration from parents or guardians is critical for supervising and recording urine excretion data at home; hence, it is important to first invite them to allow their children to participate, and to then provide clear instructions for the tasks they are expected to carry out. A clear short note of invitation should be prepared, and sent or delivered to each parent or guardian of eligible children (an example is given in Figure 3.4). Institutional review boards (IRB) or equivalent agencies oversee the safety and rights of humans who participate as research subjects. A consent form explaining the purpose and activities to be conducted, benefits and risks to subjects, participation time and other implications must be prepared by the investigators using plain language that will be easily understood by someone with limited education. IRBs require such a document to be reviewed and approved before subjects are engaged in a study. Requirements may vary from country to country, and the investigator is advised to enquire about existing requirements on this matter.

Collaboration from preschool, kindergarten or day-care centres is crucial to enable investigators to conduct studies in a smooth way. Before the day on which the urine collection is planned, it is advisable to meet with the school nurse to finalize details, identify classrooms and restroom facilities for boys and girls, and agree on the necessary project flow. Any additional information on project specifics can be provided at this time.

Collection staff

People who work closely with families, particularly in the health field, are best suited to obtaining urine collections from subjects in the survey, and are available in most countries. The key staff involved have to obtain the confidence and cooperation of subjects (and their families if relevant) and schools, supervise collection and undertake simple measurements on the urine collected.

Home kit

Collection vessel – adults and older children

Most studies are undertaken in children or adults able to control micturition. In such cases, the collection vessel is a jar or plastic bottle with a wide mouth, a lid that can be closed securely (preferably a screw cap), and an area for marking the ID. Such containers are marketed for urine collection and usually graduated in both millilitres and ounces.

The size of container required will depend on the age of the subjects; for example, children aged 3–5 years produce an average of 600–700 mL of urine in 24 hours, whereas children aged 5 years are likely to urinate more.

For collection of all urine over a 24-hourperiod:

- preschool children should be supplied with a 155-mL container; and
- older children and adults should be supplied with a 200-mL container. For nocturnal collections, a 1000-mL container may be required.

A container of 500 or 1000-mL capacity should be used for pooling urine collected from one child during one 24-hour period (the 500-mL capacity may suffice if the study includes only small children).

When urine is obtained from defined periods of a day, collection containers for use during daytime could have a capacity of 120–300 mL for each period (depending on age and the amount of liquids ingested); jars or bottles of 500-mL capacity are also appropriate.

Collection vessel – infants and young children

For infants or young children who are not toilet trained, paediatric collectors – special pants that collect all urine (referred to as a "bag within a bag") – should be used (22). The bag-within-a-bag system is designed to permit urine to flow from the inside bag to the outside bag, but not in the reverse direction; this prevents urine from being in contact with the child's genitals. The collector is provided with a wide micro pore adhesive band made of non-allergenic material to prevent skin irritation (e.g. Lil'Katch, Cat. No. 05–0501 mfg Mark Clark, Topeka, Kansas – distributed by Baxter Scientific).

Number of kits

Generally, two of the above kits are used for each subject – one for home and one for school. A third kit may be required if the subject is going somewhere else during the collection period. All items should be labelled using a waterproof marker.

Diary

A small "diary" is required and is given to the subject. The diary contains instructions, the collection supervisor's telephone number, and space for the subject (or parent) to record relevant information (see below).

Supervisor requirements

General

The collection supervisor will require the use of a small laboratory or office containing a refrigerator, a freezer, a sink, and a table or bench. The following will also be required:

- plastic measuring jug with wide neck;
- plastic funnel;
- a 1 L measuring cylinder, accurate to 10 mL;
- cold disinfecting solution; and
- 20% chlorhexidine digluconate solution, to prevent growth of microorganisms (55, 56) and reduce offensive odour; this is particularly important if pH of urine is to be determined, because growth of bacteria releases ammonia and increases the pH of the urine (56).

Labels

Labels are crucial for recording the subject's identity number. If time collections are planned, the labels may contain other information essential to the conduct of the study. A label for use specifically in time-controlled urine collections has been designed for recording personal information (Fig. 3.1), micturition times and volume for up to four time periods. This label should be firmly attached to the urine collecting jar, to ensure that it does not detach if it becomes wet during the collection process. The label should be of a size that is large enough to contain all the relevant information, but small enough to adhere securely to the jar.

If time collections are planned, a different label is used for the overnight collection (Fig. 3.2). This label includes space for entering personal information and instructions for subjects or parents, plus two recording fields.

Record book

A record book is vital – it is used to transfer and maintain a record of individual and collective data obtained by the collection supervisor in the field. The record book reduces the possibility of losing data entered in labels or forms; it can also be used for cross-referencing and verifying questionable entries. A hand-written record book is recommended because it is easier to handle.

Other essential accessories

Accessories will include a weighing scale in kilograms (one per collection site), pencils, an eraser, data-collection forms, labels (sufficient quantity), a fine-point permanent marker, disposable gloves, pens and write-on removable adhesive tape in four colours (one per period of collection). If timed collections are planned, additional equipment will be required: a 5-mL capacity graduate plastic measuring cylinder for adding 2.5 mL of 20% chlorhexidine digluconate to the urine collection bottles and a graduated 250 mL plastic cylinder for measuring urine volume at the collection site.

4 Twenty-four hour urine collection

4.1 Procedure

If it is intended to record urine pH, the collection supervisor will first add 2.5 mL of 20% chlorhexidine digluconate solution to each collection bottle.

The supervisor should visit the subject, or the subject's care taker, the day before the day of urine collection, to explain the collection procedure and give the subject a home kit and a diary. On the morning of the collection, the subject should void urine (this urine will not be collected) and record the time of this first (discarded) void in the diary. Every subsequent void should be collected. The subject should void into the wide-necked collection container and this urine should be poured into the screw-capped collection bottle, using the funnel. If possible, this collection bottle should be kept in a refrigerator.

The collection supervisor should meet the subject at school, with the second collection kit. Every time the subject wishes to pass urine, the subject and supervisor should meet to ensure complete collection and transfer of urine to the screw-cap collection bottle. If possible, this collection bottle should be kept in a refrigerator. At the end of the school day, the supervisor should collect the school kit, take it to the laboratory or office, and put the collection bottle in the refrigerator. After school, the supervisor should visit the subject at home to motivate the subject (or parent) to continue collection of urine until the first void on the next morning and remind the subject that he/she should note the time of this first void (collected urine) in the diary. In studies with adults, arrangements with the administrative superior or employer are essential.

On the following day, the supervisor should visit the subject's home to ask whether the collection was completed successfully, collect the home kit and diary, and take the collected urine to the laboratory or office. At the laboratory, all of the urine collected from the subject over the 24-hour should be poured into the 1 L measuring cylinder, and the total volume recorded. Also, the pH of the urine should be measured, if this information is required. The addition of chlorhexidine, mentioned at the beginning of this section, is essential if pH is to be determined. Small crystals of thymol can be added to the urine samples to reduce offensive odour.

Urine samples should be stored in a refrigerator, to keep them cool until they are transferred to the laboratory. If a refrigerator is not available, an insulated cooler to which ice bags or dried ice have been added can be used to keep the samples cool.

The urine should be well mixed before aliquots are taken, and the aliquots should be put in the freezer. Usually, four aliquots are taken and put into four labelled bijous: two for measurement of fluoride concentration and two for measurement of creatinine concentration. If the aliquots are to be sent by mail (or similar), it is a good idea to take two additional aliquots and store these bijous in the freezer in the laboratory or office, in case the four aliquots are lost in transit. Once the four (or six) labelled bijous are in the freezer, the remaining urine can be discarded, and the collection kits and measuring cylinder should be washed, put into disinfecting solution for the appropriate time and rinsed so that they are ready for use by the next subject.

4.2 Fluoride and creatinine concentrations

Urine aliquots intended to be used for this purpose will be conveyed to a suitable laboratory that is equipped to undertake the necessary studies (see Section 2.4.1). If possible, samples should be kept frozen during transport to the laboratory.

4.3 Information to be recorded

As noted previously, personal information must be recorded on the form and in the record book. The following must also be recorded:

- length of the collection period (from the subject's diary, recorded in decimal hours – e.g. 23.9 h, see Section 4.5 for details);
- urine pH (if needed);
- urine volume (mL), as measured;
- urine volume (mL), adjusted from recorded collection period to 24 hour;
- creatinine concentration (mg/L);
- creatinine excretion (mg/hour);
- fluoride concentration (mg/L urine or ppm); and
- fluoride excretion (mg/24 hour).

Subject data sometimes needs to be discarded. Any of the following are reasons for discarding data:

- the subject admits to incomplete collection;
- the volume of urine is outside the accepted range of volumes (see flow limits in Table 5.2, in Section 5.6); or

- the amount of creatinine excreted in urine is outside the accepted range (see Table 5.2).

For the subjects who completed the study successfully, derived data usually comprises (Table 5.1):

- number of subjects;
- gender balance (% male: female);
- age (mean, SD);
- 24-hour urine volume (mean, SD);
- fluoride concentration (mean, SD); and
- 24-hour urinary fluoride excretion (mean, SD).

4.4   Determination of fluoride in urine

Reliable methods for determining urinary fluoride concentrations are well established, and detailed procedures are given in the Appendix section: AP3.3. Procedures for determining fluoride in water obtained from the community (e.g. from the central water supply, boreholes, wells, springs, creeks or lakes) are the same as those used for determining fluoride in urine.

4.5   General rules for tabulation and processing of data

The concentration of fluoride in urine is obtained as described in Annex C or from data provided by the laboratory that conducted the fluoride determination. Whatever method is used, it is important to take into consideration essential data needed, and to comply with the following calculation rules, which provide simple numerical operations that can be performed using a basic calculator or computer programme. These rules are intended to facilitate calculation of derived data.

A. Duration of collection is calculated in hours and decimals of hour (to convert minutes to decimals of one hour, multiply by 0.01667).

B. A correction factor – obtained by dividing 24 by the actual duration of collection in a given subject – is used when the urine collection was shorter than 24 hours. The corrected volume for a subject is obtained by multiplying the recorded volume by the correction factor for that subject.

C. Quantity of fluoride in micrograms (µg) in the collected urine is obtained by multiplying urine volume (in ml) by fluoride concentration (in µg/mL; i.e. ppm).

D. Findings by kilogram of body weight and 24 hours:

a) Urine volume in mL/kg bw/day is obtained by dividing the volume of urine (in mL) in 24 hours (see point B above) by the weight of the child in kilograms.

35

b) If the investigation requires results of quantity of fluoride in µg/kg bw/day, calculations must be carried out for each child by dividing the quantity of fluoride excreted (in µg, see point C above) by the weight of the child in kilograms.

These rules are summarized in Table 7.5 in Section 7.1.

The person in charge of the assessment should obtain the average quantity of fluoride excreted in 24 hours, and compare this with the standards given in Table 5.3. If available, parameters from the shorter collection periods should be compared with the standards given in Table 7.3. These comparisons will help in deciding whether the fluoride excretion results indicate suboptimal, optimal or above optimal fluoride intake, taking into consideration the following guidelines:

- *Low fluoride intake*: fluoride up to 0.02 mg/kg bw/day (i.e. 20 µg/kg bw/day).
- *Optimal usage of fluoride*; multiple fluoride-based prevention is used, but not to an extent that would cause enamel fluorosis of cosmetic importance. The range of total optimal fluoride intake (or exposure) is 0.05–0.07 mg/kg/day (i.e. 50–70 µg/kg bw/day).

If no further data management or analyses are required, the person in charge of the study should then prepare a final report, which should include at least the information described in Section 5.

5 Design of the final report for 24-hour urine collection

This section suggests what information should be included in the various sections of a final report for a study that involved 24-hour urine collection, and how the report should be structured.

5.1 Introduction

The introduction to the report should state clearly the objectives of the study; objectives can range from surveillance of community programmes to a specific research project.

5.2 Materials and methods

The materials and methods should comply with the conventions for scientific publications, giving reasons for and methods of selecting the particular location or locations of the study, and the number and age of subjects. A separate section should provide all relevant information about the known fluoride exposure of the subjects and the population from which the subjects are drawn. For example, some traditional (mainly African) diets have been shown to be high in fluoride, whereas in industrialized countries, intensive cultivation, combined with sophisticated food processing, leads to generally low dietary fluoride content.

5.3 Results

The results section of the study report can be fairly brief, because the methods and evaluations for 24-hour collections are straightforward. Several articles provide examples of how to present the results for studies based on complete 24-hour collections (*17, 19, 21*).

The essential results of any study of this type are the 24-hour urinary fluoride excretion values, summarized when possible in the format illustrated in Table 5.1 (Section 5.6). Urinary data obtained for the purpose of this type of

Table 5.1 Urinary fluoride excretion data from 24-hour urine collections

Country/Region _____ **Location** _____
Dates: urines collected between _____ and _____

Subjects
    Number of eligible subjects _____
    Number of sampled subjects _____
    Number of subjects with consent _____
    Number of subjects with complete collections _____
    Mean (and SD) age _____
    Mean (and SD) weight (kg) _____

Duration of collection, (hours) within one 24-hour cycle
    Mean (and SD) _____

Urine volume (mL) per 24-hour cycle
    Mean (and SD)
    Confidence range (95%)

Urine volume (mL) per kg bw per 24-hour cycle
    Mean (and SD)
    Confidence range (95%)

Fluoride concentration (mg/L)
    Mean (and SD)
    Confidence range (95%)

Fluoride excretion (µg) per 24-hour cycle
    Mean (and SD)
    Confidence range (95%)

Fluoride excretion (µg) per kg bw per 24-hour cycle
    Mean (and SD)
    Confidence range (95%)

Fluoride excretion (µg) per hour
    Mean (and SD)
    Confidence range (95%)

bw, body weight; SD, standard deviation

study tend to be skewed; therefore, frequency distributions presented as histograms or in tabular form are useful, because they allow the maximum amount of information to be extracted from the data.

If the pH of urine has been measured (e.g. if the community is known to consume a diet high in either meat or vegetable, as discussed in Section 1.3), the results of pH values would be recorded, and used to aid interpretation of the findings.

5.4   Discussion and conclusion

As with scientific articles, the discussion should contain four topics:

- a brief statement of the main findings;
- a critique of the methods used;
- a discussion of how the findings fit with previous or published information; and
- a discussion of the implications of the findings, and suggestions for further investigation.

Table 5.3 provides standards of urinary fluoride excretion in 24-hour urine collections associated with low fluoride exposure and for the range of "optimal" exposure to fluoride, which is 0.05–0.07 mg/kg bw/day.

If the study is designed to determine existing levels of fluoride exposure before introduction of a fluoride programme, the fluoride excretion data gathered should be related to any available information about local sources of fluoride. In follow-up studies (1 month after implementation of a milk fluoridation programme or 9 months after implementation of water or salt fluoridation), conclusions should indicate whether urinary fluoride findings are low, high, or optimal in relation to the standards given in Table 7.3 for timed collection studies.

5.5   Summary

The summary should describe the purpose of the study, sources of fluoride exposure and the main findings. It could include suggestions for intensifying an existing fluoridation programme in order to achieve maximum benefits, or reducing fluoride exposure to avoid detrimental effects, as appropriate.

5.6 Tables for the 24-hour collection method

Table 5.2 Criteria for cleaning data from children aged 2–6 years, from 24-hour collections

	Urinary flow	
	Lower limit	**Upper limit**
Age 2–4 years (mL/24 hours)	140	–
Age 4–6 years (mL/24 hours)	200	–
Age 2–4 years (mL/hour)	5	–
Age 4–6 years (mL/hour)	7	–

24-hour urinary excretion of creatinine

	Urinary creatinine (mg/kg bw/day)[a]	
Age (year)	**Male**	**Female**
<1	8–20	8–20
1–11	8–22	8–22
12–15	8–30	8–30
16–89	14–26	11–20
≥90	>9	>9

Urinary recovery of PABA[b]
In relation to urinary recovery of PABA, complete urinary collections are those with urinary recovery of PABA of 85–110%

bw, body weight; PABA, para-aminobenzoic acid
a Indicators of incomplete collections are urine samples with <8 mg creatinine/kg bw/day; Indicators of collections of >24 hours are urine samples with >22 mg creatinine/kg bw/day
b Subjects are given 80 mg PABA tablets, to be taken at specified intervals with meals. Completeness is then assessed by measuring urinary recovery of PABA over 24 hours

Table 5.3 Standards for urinary fluoride excretion (mg/24-hour cycle): lower and upper margins

Low exposure to fluoride (intake <0.02 mg per 24-hour cycle)	Range of optimal fluoride intake	
	Lower margin[a]	Upper margin[b]
Age 2–4 years, approximate bw 15.3 kg		
≤0.14	0.30	0.41
Age 3–5 years, approximate bw 17.3 kg		
≤0.15	0.33	0.45
Age 4–6 years, approximate bw 19.2 kg		
≤0.16	0.37	0.50
Age 10–14 years, approximate bw 43.1 kg		
≤0.33	0.79	1.10

bw, body weight
a Lower margin based on a fluoride intake of 0.05 mg/kg bw/day
b Upper margin based on a fluoride intake of 0.07 mg/kg bw/say
Note: For calculations, see Tables 5.4 and 5.5

Table 5.4 Calculated daily urinary fluoride excretion associated with low, optimal and high fluoride intake for ages 1–14 years

Age at last birthday	Age range		Exact age	Mean weight	Exposure multiplied by bw				Calculated DUFE			
	Minimal	Maximal			Low exposure (0.02 mgF/kg × bw)	Optimal range		High exposure (0.1 mgF/kg × bw)	Low exposure (0.02 mgF/kg)	Optimal range 0.05–0.07 mgF/kg		High exposure (0.1 mgF/kg)
						0.05 mgF/kg × bw	0.07 mgF/kg × bw			0.05 mgF/kg	0.07 mgF/kg	
Yrs	Months	Months	Yrs	kg[a]	"Too low"	Lower limit	Upper limit	"Too high"	mg/24 h	mg/24 h	mg/24 h	mg/24 h
1	12	23	1.5	11.1	0.222	0.555	0.777	1.110	0.108	0.224	0.302	0.419
2	24	35	2.5	13.3	0.266	0.665	0.931	1.330	0.123	0.263	0.356	0.496
3	36	47	3.5	15.4	0.308	0.770	1.078	1.540	0.138	0.300	0.407	0.569
4	48	59	4.5	17.3	0.346	0.865	1.211	1.730	0.151	0.333	0.454	0.636
5	60	71	5.5	19.1	0.382	0.955	1.337	1.910	0.164	0.364	0.498	0.699
6	72	83	6.5	21.2	0.424	1.060	1.484	2.120	0.178	0.401	0.549	0.772
7	84	95	7.5	22.3	0.446	1.115	1.561	2.230	0.186	0.420	0.576	0.811
8	96	107	8.5	25.1	0.502	1.255	1.757	2.510	0.206	0.469	0.645	0.909
9	108	119	9.5	28.2	0.564	1.410	1.974	2.820	0.227	0.524	0.721	1.017
10	120	131	10.5	34.0	0.680	1.70	2.38	3.40	0.268	0.625	0.863	1.220
11	132	143	11.5	38.3	0.766	1.92	2.68	3.83	0.298	0.700	0.968	1.371
12	144	155	12.5	43.1	0.862	2.16	3.02	4.31	0.332	0.784	1.086	1.539
13	156	167	13.5	48.0	0.960	2.40	3.36	4.80	0.366	0.870	1.206	1.710
14	168	179	14.5	52.9	1.058	2.65	3.70	5.29	0.400	0.956	1.326	1.882

bw, body weight; DUFE, daily urinary fluoride excretion; F, fluoride; h, hour; TDFI, total daily fluoride intake; yr, year
Note: DUFE = TDFI × 0.35 + 0.03 [Villa et al. (2010), (17), equation 1]
a Bodyweight according to United States National Center for Health Statistics

Table 5.5 Calculated daily urinary fluoride excretion associated with low, optimal and high fluoride intake for broader age groups

Age at last birthday	Age range		Exact age	Mean weight	Exposure multiplied by bw				Calculated DUFE			
	Minimal	Maximal			Low exposure (0.02 mgF/kg × bw)	Optimal range		High exposure (0.1 mgF/kg × bw)	Low exposure (0.02 mgF/kg)	Optimal range		High exposure (0.1 mgF/kg)
						0.05 mgF/kg × bw	0.07 mgF/kg × bw			0.05 mgF/kg	0.07 mgF/kg	
Years	Months	Months	Yrs	In kg[a]	"Too low"	Lower limit	Upper limit	"Too high"	mg/24hrs	mg/24h	mg/24h	mg/24 hours
	Age range in months											
1–2	12	35	2.0	12.2	0.244	0.610	0.854	1.220	0.115	0.244	0.329	0.457
2–3	24	47	3.0	14.4	0.287	0.718	1.005	1.435	0.130	0.281	0.382	0.532
3–4	36	59	4.0	16.4	0.327	0.818	1.145	1.635	0.144	0.316	0.431	0.602
4–5	48	71	5.0	18.2	0.364	0.910	1.274	1.820	0.157	0.349	0.476	0.667
5–6	60	83	6.0	20.2	0.403	1.008	1.411	2.015	0.171	0.383	0.524	0.735
6–7	72	95	7.0	21.8	0.435	1.008	1.523	2.175	0.182	0.411	0.563	0.791
1–3	12	47	2.5	13.3	0.265	0.663	0.929	1.327	0.123	0.262	0.355	0.494
2–4	24	59	3.5	15.3	0.307	0.767	1.073	1.533	**0.137**	**0.298**	**0.406**	0.567
3–5	36	71	4.5	17.3	0.345	0.863	1.209	1.727	**0.151**	**0.332**	**0.453**	0.634
4–6	48	83	5.5	19.2	0.384	0.960	1.344	1.920	**0.164**	**0.366**	**0.500**	0.702
5–7	60	95	6.5	20.9	0.417	1.043	1.461	2.087	0.176	0.395	0.541	0.760
1–4	12	59	3.0	14.3	0.286	0.714	0.999	1.428	0.130	0.280	0.380	0.530
2–5	24	71	4.0	16.3	0.326	0.814	1.139	1.628	0.144	0.315	0.429	0.600
3–6	36	83	5.0	18.3	0.365	0.913	1.278	1.825	0.158	0.349	0.477	0.669
4–7	48	95	6.0	20.0	0.400	0.999	1.398	1.998	0.170	0.380	0.519	0.729
1–5	12	71	3.5	15.2	0.305	0.762	1.067	1.524	0.137	0.297	0.403	0.563
2–6	24	83	4.5	17.3	0.345	0.863	1.208	1.726	0.151	0.332	0.453	0.634
3–7	48	95	5.5	19.1	0.381	0.953	1.334	1.906	0.163	0.364	0.497	0.697
1–6	12	83	4.0	16.2	0.325	0.812	1.136	1.623	0.144	0.314	0.428	0.598
2–7	24	95	5.0	18.1	0.362	0.905	1.267	1.810	0.157	0.347	0.473	0.664
1–7	12	95	4.5	17.1	0.342	0.855	1.197	1.710	0.150	0.329	0.449	0.629
10–14	120	173	12.5	43.3	0.865	2.163	3.028	4.326	**0.333**	**0.787**	**1.090**	1.544

bw, body weight; DUFE, daily urinary fluoride excretion; h, hour; TDFI, total daily fluoride intake; yr, year

Notes: DUFE = TDFI*0.35 + 0.03 [Villa et al. (2010); (17), equation 1]; the figures in bold fonts in columns10, 11 and 12 were used for Table 5.3

a Body weight according to United States National Center for Health Statistics

6 Collections of 8–18 hours (within the 24-hour cycle)

Any urine collection must cover a period of at least 2 hours. Incomplete voiding of the bladder at the start or end of the collection period should be avoided, because it can significantly affect the results. To ensure that the total urine generated during the specified period is collected, the procedure involves recording the time at which the collection began and ended (in hours and minutes), and the volume of urine collected as outlined below:

- At the beginning of each collection period, ensure that the subject empties his or her bladder completely:
  — If this is the first collection taken from the subject, discard this urine.
  — If this micturition is the end of a collection period, add the urine passed at this time to the jar used to collect the previous samples from that collection period.
- Note the name of the subject and the time in box No. 1 of the respective period on the label or in the record book (see Fig. 3.1).
- When the subject arrives for the next urination, give the subject the jar or container into which they are to urinate.
- Note the time of this second urination. Ensure that the jar or container is closed, and then put in a cool place (e.g. a refrigerator). If no refrigerator is available, an insulated cooler to which ice bags or dried ice have been added can be used to keep the urine cool before it is transferred to the laboratory. Handle the next and any subsequent urination in the same pre-set collection period in an identical manner.

Towards the end of the supervised pre-set collection period, ask the subject to urinate into the jar. The time when this takes place marks the end of the subject's personal period.

- Measure the total volume of urine collected during this period using a graduated plastic cylinder 250 mL capacity (or cylinders of 100 or 500 mL capacity can be used, if available), and note the volume on the label and in the record book.

At this point, the base information available from each subject is:

- time point of initial voiding of the bladder;
- time point of last urine collection into the container (jar or bottle); and
- total volume of urine collected between initial and final time points.

For the purpose of analysis, take a 15–25 mL sample of urine from each jar into in a small tube. If possible, take additional aliquots as a safeguard against loss of urine. Store the tubes in a container containing ice for transfer to the laboratory. If fluoride determination cannot be conducted immediately, place tubes in a freezer at –18°C or in a refrigerator, if no freezer are available. Ensure that all tubes are labelled with a reference number that identifies the individual from whom the sample came, and the time period in which the sample was collected. It is good practice to colour code the collection periods (A, B, C or D), mark each tube with the subject ID number using the fine-point permanent ink marker, and also identify the location of the collection.

Wherever possible, obtain a night collection and two supervised day collections. Typically, a night collection in children is obtained under parental supervision and covers 8–10 hours. The two daytime collections are made under supervision of teachers, and one or two members of the project team. Each daytime collection should last about 3–5 hours. In this way, a total of 14–18 hours of the entire 24-hour cycle will be covered. As noted above, in some countries it may only be possible to obtain a morning and a nocturnal collection; these would total 12–15 hours.

6.1 Collection of nocturnal urine and during periods of high excretion

A specific jar with a capacity of 750–800 mL is used for a nocturnal collection; with children, this collection is made under parental supervision. A sample label for a nocturnal collection is depicted in Fig. 3.2. Instruct parents to note the time at which the child urinates before going to bed, or the adult participant to note the time at which he/she urinated before going to bed, and advise them not to collect that urine in the jar. If the child or adult participant needs to urinate during the night he or she should use the jar. When the jar is brought in the next morning, measure the volume of urine and record it both on the label and in the record book. In adults, cooperation may sometimes be difficult to obtain. In cases of doubt, it may be advisable to choose another person.

The summary data can be entered in the form prepared for this purpose (Fig. 3.3) and in the record book. A spreadsheet created using Microsoft (MS) Excel software can be used for entering data and calculating results (Tables 7.6 and 7.7). These data are entered in columns 12–14, 22–24 and 32–34, and are used to in calculating fluoride excretion per time.

Generally, fluoride excretion is highest 1–2 hours after the main cooked meal, and lowest during the night; morning urine is also low in fluoride. Accordingly, the two columns to the left in Table 7.3 show the lower and upper margins for high excretion periods (e.g. after intake of fluoridated milk, meals prepared with fluoridated salt, or consumption of high-fluoride mineral water or some other fluoride source). The two columns to the right in Table 7.3 show the lower and upper margins for urine not preceded – for at least 3 hours – by significant fluoride intake.

6.2 Optional calculations obtained from time-controlled urine collection – Use of a standardized format

The question whether or not urinary fluoride excretion in a given population is at the desired level can be answered by straightforward evaluation of 24-hour urine collections. The calculations are simple, but it is vital to record all factors that may affect individual and group outcomes. This method has been carried over from the first edition of the manual on monitoring of renal fluoride excretion (*11*), and is intended to assist those interested in obtaining a more comprehensive evaluation of results of renal fluoride excretion using MS Excel (Sections 1.0–3.2.1 of this document apply).

A standard format is presented in Table 7.6 (see Section 7.1), to illustrate the recording and evaluation of field and laboratory data. This format was developed and extensively tested under various working conditions. Sources of data on fluoride intake or exposure should be entered in rows 1 and 2 of the spreadsheet. A simple coding system should be designed to facilitate data entry (see Section 6.2.1 below). For direct comparison with other data, two columns with 24-hour results shown on a per-hour basis have been included (columns 21 and 22).

Some general rules must be followed for appropriate processing of data using the standard format described above. Following such rules will make it easier to process the data, and will thus help to reduce errors and frustration. Data are entered as hours and minutes – using no commas, full stops or colons (e.g. 715 and 630); and midnight must be recorded as 2400 rather than 0000, because any value equal to 0 in any of the columns 11–14 renders the data for a collection invalid.

Precision in recording time is essential. In 24-hour collections, time should be recorded to the nearest quarter of an hour (15 minutes); in shorter collections, it should be recorded to the nearest 5 minutes or 1 minute. Entries must be in the format "hhmm" (i.e. with no decimal point) for the time of initial voiding and final collection. Volume of urine should be determined to the nearest 5 mL in 24-hour collections, but to the nearest 2 mL in shorter collection periods. Measuring cylinders for up to 250 mL usually have 2 mL divisions; whereas those for up to 500 mL have 5 mL divisions.

Fluoride concentrations should be recorded with two digits after the decimal point (e.g. 0.65 ppm). In the case of low concentrations, three decimal places may be provided by the laboratory. Figures that include three decimal places (e.g. 0.095 ppm) should not be rounded up. The computed values (columns 15 and above) are calculated by the computer using at least six decimals (floating point operations). The format of the depicted values is specified in the programmed part of the tables and does not alter the high precision of the calculations.

6.2.1   *Coded recordings of personal data and individual fluoride exposure*

In Tables 7.6–7.8, the titles and column headings are self-explanatory (these occupy rows 1–9 in the MS Excel spreadsheet). Column numbers are given below the headings (in row 10). Data for the first subject are then recorded in row 11, for the second subject in row 12, and so on. Thus, if a study involves 37 subjects, data for the last subject will occupy row 47. In MS Excel, the rows are numbered, making it easier to check the data in studies involving large numbers of subjects. Columns are used in a similarly systematic manner; with columns 1–10 reserved for personal information (see Section 3.1.2).

Column 1	The subject ID number (not necessarily in strict sequential order, unless the investigator has rearranged the spreadsheet to cross-reference with the code number; this extra step is not recommended because it is unnecessary, and creates room for errors).
Column 2	Gender (male = 1 and female = 2)
Column 3	Age in years at last birthday
Column 4	Body weight in kilograms
Columns 5–10	Coded data on individual fluoride intake or fluoride exposure, and other relevant information
Column 5	Use of fluoridated milk or salt: No = 0; Yes = 1
Column 6	Use of fluoride-containing toothpaste: Never = 0; Sometimes = 1; Once a day = 1; At least twice a day = 3
Column 7	Amount of toothpaste used by child: Small pea size = 1; Half of the toothbrush length =2; Entire length of the toothbrush = 3
Column 8	Who places the toothpaste on the child's toothbrush: The child = 1; The mother or another relative = 2
Column 9	Does the mother or an adult person supervise the child during tooth brushing? Yes = 1; No = 2

| Column 10 | Use of prescribed or over-the-counter fluoride supplements: Never = 0; Sometimes = 1; Daily = 2 |
| Column 11 | Repeats Column 1, and pertains to the block of columns 11–20 |

6.2.2 Standard table for surveys with 24-hour collections

It is important to take into consideration the format to be used for entering time data. As explained in Section 6.2.1, the time of day at which the collection is initiated and the time at which it ends is expressed in hours and minutes using no commas, full stops or colons. The duration of the collection is expressed in hours and decimals hours; conversion to this format is essential for subsequent arithmetic procedures. Because it is difficult to obtain an exact 24-hour collection, a correction factor is calculated, and is then used to obtain the corrected 24-hour urinary volume and fluoride excretion (see Section 4.5).

In Table 7.6, field and laboratory data (i.e. data at the beginning and end of the collection period, urine volume and fluoride concentration) are entered in columns 12–15:

Column 12	Time at the start of urine collection (hhmm); that is, the time at which the subject emptied his or her bladder (this urine is not time-controlled, and is therefore discarded unless it pertains to and terminates a preceding collection)
Column 13	Time of final micturition into the container
Column 14	Volume (mL) of urine
Column 15	Fluoride concentration (ppm)

The data that must be entered into the table are shown in italics, and contained within two frames (covering columns 1–10 and 12–15). As an example, Table 7.6 has been completed for six subjects to illustrate how the table should be used.

Results computed from the field and laboratory data in columns 12–15 are presented in columns 16–24:

| Column 16 | Duration in hh. decimals of the collection; thus, for subject 1 in the example, duration is 23.25 hours (i.e. 23 hours 15 minutes) |
| Column 17 | Quantity (in µg) of fluoride in the urine collection, obtained by multiplying the value in column 14 by that in column 15; thus, for subject 4 in the example, the quantity of fluoride is $600 \times 0.4 = 240$ |

Column 18	Correction factor to yield exact 24-hour values, obtained by dividing 24 by the duration of collection (Column 16); thus, for subject 4 in the example, the factor is $24/24.67 = 0.973$
Column 19	Corrected 24-hour urinary volume in mL, obtained by multiplying the volume collected (column 14) by the correction factor (column 18); thus, for subject 2 in the example, who collected 710 mL of urine, the corrected volume is $710 \times 0.973 = 691$ mL
Column 20	Corrected 24-hour fluoride excretion (in µg), obtained by multiplying the quantity of fluoride in the urine actually collected (column 17) by the correction factor (column 18); thus, for subject 2 in the example, the corrected fluoride excretion is $256 \text{ µg} \times 0.973 = 249$ µg
Column 21	Urinary flow in mL/hour, obtained by dividing the value in column 19 – corrected 24-hour urinary volume in mL – by 24
Column 22	Hourly urinary fluoride excretion, obtained by dividing the value in column 20 – corrected 24-hour fluoride excretion (in µg) – by 24; hourly values are useful for comparison with results of studies limited to certain parts of the 24-hour period
Column 23	24-hour urinary volume per kilogram body weight, obtained by dividing the value in column 19 by that entered in column 4 (i.e. subject weight in kg)
Column 24	24-hour urinary fluoride excretion per kilogram body weight, obtained by dividing the value in column 20 – corrected 24-hour fluoride excretion in µg – by that entered in column 4 (subject weight in kg)

Basic statistics are displayed automatically below each column that shows data for individual subjects. Minimum and maximum values are given, and must always be examined to identify "outliers", which may result from mis-reporting or methodological errors (see Section 6.2.6). Median values and arithmetic mean values are also given; median values are generally slightly lower than the mean values because it is quite common for very high values to be obtained from a few individuals, resulting in a skewed distribution. Values for SD, CV and standard error are also presented.

In studies of circadian variations, it may be convenient to collect and separately analyse 24-hour urine in two (day and night), three or even four separate periods. In such cases, Table 7.6 cannot be used. These data are more complicated to handle; the amount of fluoride in the collection, for instance, must be computed for each time period rather than being averaged over the periods.

Tables are available for use with these data, using the same format shown in columns 1–10, 12–15, 22–25, etc. (see Section 6.2).

6.2.3   Standard table for surveys with two collections totalling 14–16 hours, using MS Excel

As in Table 7.6, columns 1–10 of Table 7.7 are reserved for personal data and codes relating to individual fluoride exposure, and column 11 repeats the subject number. For the *first collection period*, columns 12–15 are again used for recording field and laboratory data, with the same use of italics and boxes as in Table 7.6. In the example given, except for two children, the first collection took place during the night; results for this period are given in columns 16–20.

Column 16	Validity code. If the initial time, the final time, the volume and the fluoride concentration of the collection (columns 12–15) are available, the code 1 – "valid" – appears in column 16. If one or more of these values are missing, the code in column 16 is 0, indicating an "unsuccessful" collection. Missing data could be due to the initial or final time of the collection (or both) being missing, the collected urine being lost, or the fluoride concentration being unavailable. As noted above, midnight must be recorded as 2400, not as 0000, because any value equal to 0 in any of the columns 12–15 renders the data for a collection invalid. Whenever the code in column 16 is 0, an "**x**" is automatically assigned to columns 17–20.
Column 17	Time of initial voiding (column 12). This is recorded only for those children whose urine collection was successful. The median time at the start of the collections is important when comparing fluoride excretion with a distinct time point of fluoride, as in Table 7.3.
Column 18	Duration of collection, expressed in hours and decimals (hh.dec). The underlying formula automatically takes into account the special situation of collections extending past midnight; when the initial time of a collection is a larger figure – for example, if the collection ran from 2200 (i.e. 10 pm) to 0700 (i.e. 7 am) – then 24 hours are automatically added to the final time; this gives the correct duration, which in the case of this example would be 9 hours.

Column 19	Urinary flow (mL/hour)
Column 20	Urinary fluoride excretion (µg/hour)
Column 21	Subject number(automatically presented)

Data from the *second collection period* are entered in columns 22–25 of Table 7.6: columns 26–31 then correspond exactly to columns 16–21; that is, they cover the validity code, time of initial voiding, duration of collection, urinary flow, urinary excretion rate and subject number. The data for the fifth subject (No. 85) have been processed to illustrate the ease of the computations.

The statistics on the fluoride excretion shown in column 20 (nocturnal collections) should be compared to the standards given in Table 7.3.

6.2.4 Standard table for surveys with three collections totalling 14–16 hours using MS Excel: complete series

The term "complete series" applies when all the three collections are valid in all subjects, and can thus be evaluated in respective tables. In Table 7.7, only seven subjects provided complete data; 2 subjects (Nos. 84 and 87) provided only noon data, and one subject (No. 91) provided no valid data at all.

When three collection periods are chosen – for example, morning, midday and nocturnal urine – the morning results are entered in columns 12–21, the midday results in columns 22–31, and the nocturnal data and respective results in columns 32–41.

Under Westernized eating habits, the nocturnal and morning results should be compared with the standards for the low excretion period, whereas the midday urine should be compared with the high excretion periods.

6.2.5 Standard table for surveys with collections made in four periods totalling the 24-cycle

The table for three collections (Section 6.2.4) must be extended by columns 42–51. This pattern of collecting urine has been used for very young children in order to identify whether there are strong circadian variations in the fluoride excretion at very young age. Studies using four collections may also be interesting in closed institutions for children.

6.2.6 Cleaning of data

When all data have been entered in the appropriate table, and all parameters have been computed (automatically for the most part), the next step is to clean the data. This process begins with inspection of the minimum and maximum values, displayed in all tables in the two rows immediately below the row that records the number of subjects.

In surveys where collections are for 14–16 hours or 8 hours, data cleaning must be done carefully, and additional criteria may need to be established. For instance, the protocol may require that, for nocturnal urine collection in children, the last urine before sleep must be passed between 19.00 and midnight, and the first morning urine between 05.00 and 09.00. Thus, if a nocturnal collection starts at 18.30, for example, it would be excluded according to these limits. However, in some societies, children (particularly those aged over 4–5 years) may not go to bed so early, so their last micturition before going to bed may occur, for example, at 21.00. Similarly, these children may get up in the morning at 6.00 or 6.30, and their first urination time would constitute the end of the nocturnal collection. Any such criteria for data cleaning must be adapted to the local customs and circumstances; these should be established during the planning stage and clearly stated in the protocol.

The minimum and maximum values shown just below the number of subjects immediately reveal "suspect" data or values that are obviously outside expected limits. Suggested limits for urinary flow, fluoride excretion rate and fluoride concentration are given in Table 7.2. When there are suspect results, the subject should be identified and the original record examined to determine whether there was a typing error, or whether something went wrong with the collection or the laboratory analysis. Only typing mistakes and obvious gross errors should be corrected in the original data table; other suspect data should be left unchanged, and no further changes should be made to this original data table. However, a copy – the "clean data table" – should be made on which suspect or doubtful data in columns 11–24, 21–24 and so on (i.e. the results that deviate significantly from normal or expected values) can be "cleaned". Although incomplete voiding of the bladder has no influence on concentrations, time-controlled samples are susceptible to incomplete voiding at the beginning and at the end of the collection period; this is the principal source of "outliers" with very high or very low urinary flow.

Cleaning of outliers must be done cautiously, and should be restricted to results that are obviously incompatible with the rest of the data. If a decision is made to exclude a particular set of results, only the initial time is to be deleted; entries in columns 15–19, 25–29 and so on will then automatically be changed to an "x". The effect of such exclusion is easy to check by comparing statistics based on the uncleaned data (in the *original* data table) with those based on the cleaned data (in the *clean* data table) Clearly, maximum and minimum values will change when outliers are excluded, but averages and medians should change very little. SD values may decrease appreciably as a result of exclusions.

In studies in which three collection series have been planned, provided that more than 80% of the children still have three valid collections in the *clean* data table, data for the children who provided complete collections may be transferred to a table designated for children with all three collections. By doing this, data for any children who provided incomplete collections are disregarded.

6.3 Extrapolations

As noted under Section 2.4.1, in some highly industrialized and in some developing countries it is not feasible to undertake collections lasting 24 hours. In these circumstances, supervised urine collection can only be taken, for instance, during the morning and the afternoon or evening, or during the morning and during nocturnal periods. However, this can give a total of 16 hours, which would mean excretion was measured during two thirds of the cycle (i.e. 16/24 hours). If one collection is timed to occur during maximal fluoride excretion and the other during low excretion (usually the nocturnal urine), then it is tempting to extrapolate from the 16-hour results to 24-hour results. Two published studies have used a simple method for such extrapolations (*43, 47*). Although the results of these studies looked "reasonable", more research is needed in this field, and it is best at this time to compare the observed results in the various collection periods with the standards given in Table 5.4.

7 Design of the final report for time-controlled urinary collections

The suggestions given in Section 5 for preparing a final report for surveys with a 24-hour collection should be considered when developing reports for surveys of a shorter duration. When the 24-hour period is subdivided, the results should be presented separately for the defined periods of the 24-hour cycle [e.g. see (57)]. The results should be presented in detail, and in a way that allows the reader to follow the calculations. For 24-hour collections, Table 7.6 presents a base table using MS Excel; such a table may be placed in an annex to the report. Table 7.7 shows an appropriate MS Excel table for studies using a nocturnal and a daytime collection; again, this table may be placed in an annex. Table 7.8 presents a dataset example and MS Excel computing table showing calculations of fluoride excretion of children providing morning, afternoon and nocturnal collections. Tables of this kind are the important outcome of timed urinary fluoride excretion studies.

Table 7.3 provides standards for urinary fluoride excretion in micrograms of fluoride per hour, which are applicable to timed collections during the 2–4 hours after the main meal, and for night and morning urinary collections. Table 7.4 provides standards for urinary fluoride concentration for communities with low fluoride intake and those with optimal fluoride intake. Table 7 displays the calculation of parameters using simple numerical operations.

7.1 Tables for time-controlled urinary collections

Table 7.1 Urinary fluoride data for time-controlled urine collections

Country/Region _____
Location _____
Dates Urines collected between _____ and _____

Number of subjects			
Eligible subjects	____	____	____
Sampled subjects	____	____	____
Subjects with consent	____	____	____
Subjects with complete collections	____	____	____
Mean (and SD) age	____	____	____
Mean (and SD) weight (kg)	____	____	____

	Period 1 (High)	Period 2 (Low)	Period 3 (Nocturnal)
Duration of collection (hours)	____	____	____
Mean (and SD)	____	____	____
(Average in hours and decimals of hour)			
Approximate beginning of the period	____	____	____
Urine volume (mL)			
Mean (and SD)	____	____	____
Confidence range (95%)	____	____	____
Urine volume (mL) per hour			
Mean (and SD)	____	____	____
Confidence range (95%)	____	____	____
Fluoride concentration (mg/L)			
Mean (and SD)	____	____	____
Confidence range (95%)	____	____	____
Fluoride excretion (μg) per kg body weight			
Mean (and SD)	____	____	____
Confidence range (95%)	____	____	____
Fluoride excretion (μg) per hour			
Mean (and SD)	____	____	____
Confidence range (95%)	____	____	____

SD, standard deviation

Table 7.2 Criteria for cleaning data from children aged 2–6 years, from time-controlled urine collections[a]

Initiation and ending of urine collection periods
Morning urine collection
First urine must be collected between 05:00 and 09:00

Nocturnal urine collection
Last urine before sleep must be passed between 19.00 and midnight

	Lower limits	Upper limits
Urinary flow		
Age 2–4 years (mL/hour)	5	____
Age 4–6 years (mL/hour)	7	____
Age 2–4 years (mL/24 hours)	140	____
Age 4–6 years (mL/24 hours)	200	____
Urinary fluoride excretion		
Age 2–4 years (μg/hour)	2	180
Age 4–6 years (μg /hour)	3	300
Age 2–4 years (mg/24 hours)	0.12	4
Age 4–6 years (mg/24 hours)	0.20	7
Urinary fluoride concentration		
All ages mg/L (ppm)	0.08	5

Note: Although incomplete voiding of the bladder has no influence on concentrations, time-controlled samples are susceptible to incomplete voiding at the beginning and at the end of the collection period; this is the principal source of "outliers" with very high or very low urinary flow

Note for the printer: μg/hour means: micrograms/hour

a Fluoride data from Bulgaria (mainly for low fluoride limits); England; Islamic Republic of Iran (mainly for high fluoride limits); Sri Lanka and Switzerland

Table 7.3 Range of optimal urinary fluoride excretion (μg/hour) at different times, for time-controlled urine collections: lower and upper margins

Optimal for peaks 2–4 hours after main meal[a]		Optimal for night and morning[b]	
Lower margin	Upper margin	Lower margin	Upper margin
Age, 2–4 years, approximate body weight 15.3 kg			
19	25	9	13
Age, 3–5 years, approximate body weight 17.3 kg			
21	28	10	14
Age, 4–6 years, approximate body weight 19.2 kg			
23	31	11	16
Age 10–14 years, approximate body weight 43.1 kg			
49	68	25	34

a 50% higher than 24-hour average
b 25% lower than 24-hour average
Note: For calculations, see Tables 5.4 and 5.5

Table 7.4 Standards for urinary fluoride concentration (mg/L; ppm) for all ages, for time-controlled urine collections; lower and upper margins

Fluoride intake	Peaks 2–4 hours after main meal		Night and morning	
	Lower limit	Upper limit	Lower limit	Upper limit
Low intake	0.3	0.5	0.2	0.4
Optimal usage[a]	0.8	1.2	0.7	0.9

a Based on large number of studies in communities with low fluoride intake and with optimal fluoride intake (mostly conducted in relation to fluoridated water), these limits have been found to be age independent

Table 7.5 Calculation of parameters using simple numerical operations

	Duration of collection in hours and decimals of hour[a]	Correction for urine collection lasting <24 hours[b]	Corrected volume (mL)	Quantity of fluoride in urine collection (μg)	Urine volume (mL/kgbw/day)	Fluoride (iμg/kg/bw/day)[c]
Relevant part of Section 4.5	A	B	B	C	D(a)	D(b)
Operation	Time at end of collection minus time at beginning of collection	Actual duration of collection, divided by 24	Recorded volume of urine (in mL) multiplied by the correction factor for that subject	Volume of urine (in mL) multiplied by fluoride concentration (in μg/mL; ppm)	Volume of urine (in mL) in 24 hours (B) divided by the weight of the child (in kg)	Quantity of fluoride excreted (in μg) [C] divided by the weight of the child (in kg)

bw, body weight; ppm, parts per million

a Minutes are multiplied by 0.01667 to convert to decimals of one hour

b A correction factor is used when the urine collection did not last exactly 24 hours

c Calculations are carried out for each child

Table 7.6 Data and computing table using MS Excel for surveys for 24-hour collections (example with six cases)

F exposure Continued — Six cases for illustration, corresponding to low or moderate fluoride exposure
(This is also for description of general fluoride intake/exposure). See case 4 with "easy" results illustrating computations

Column groupings:
- **Personal data, fluoride exposure:** Cn1–Cn11 (Cn5–Cn10 = Coded individual F exposure, etc.: F-water, F-toothpaste, F-rinses)
- **Field and laboratory data:**
  - Urine collection: Cn12–Cn15
  - Preliminary results: Cn16–Cn18
  - Correction factor for 24 h: Cn18
  - Results adjusted to 24 h: Cn19–Cn20
  - 24-h results per h: Cn21–Cn22
  - Findings per kg bw and per 24 h: Cn23–Cn24

Cn1	Cn2	Cn3	Cn4	Cn5	Cn6	Cn7	Cn8	Cn9	Cn10	Cn11	Cn12	Cn13	Cn14	Cn15	Cn16	Cn17	Cn18	Cn19	Cn20	Cn21	Cn22	Cn23	Cn24
Subject ID	Sex M=1 F=2	Age (yrs)	Bw (kg)	F-water	F-toothpaste	F-rinses				No.	Time at initial voiding (hhmm)	Collection ended (hhmm)	Volume urine mL	F conc. (ppm)	Duration of collect. (hhmm)	F in urine (µg)	Correction factor for 24h	Volume of urine (mL/24h)	F excreted (µg/24h)	Urine (mL/h)	F excreted (µg/h)	Urine (mL/kgbw/24h)	F (mg/kg/24h)
1	2	5	21	1							715	630	660	0.52	23.25	343	1.032	681	354	28.4	14.8	32.4	16.9
2	2	4	15	2							720	800	710	0.36	24.67	256	0.973	691	249	28.8	10.4	46.1	16.6
4	1	4	20	2							715	715	600	0.4	24.00	240	1.000	600	240	25.0	10.0	30.0	12.0
5	2	5	23	0							730	700	390	0.38	23.50	148	1.021	398	151	16.6	6.3	17.3	6.6
7	1	4	18	2							700	730	840	0.54	24.50	454	0.980	823	444	34.3	18.5	45.7	24.7
9	1	4	22	1							750	750	1070	0.283	24.17	303	0.993	1063	301	44.3	12.5	48.2	13.7
N	6	6	6							6			6	6	6	6	6	6	6	6	6	6	6
Min		4	15.0								700	630	390	0.283	23.25	148	0.973	398	151	16.6	6.3	17.3	6.6
Max		5	23.0								740	800	1070	0.540	24.67	454	1.032	1063	444	44.3	18.5	48.3	24.7
Med		4	20.5								717.5	732.5	685	0.390	24.08	279	0.997	686	275	28.6	11.4	39.1	15.1
Mean		4.3	19.8										712	0.414	24.01	291	1.000	709	290	29.6	12.1	36.6	15.1
SD		0.5	2.9										230	0.099	0.55	103	0.023	222	101	9.3	4.2	12.2	6.0
CV													32	24	2	36	2	31	35	31	3.5	3.3	4.0
SE													94	0.040	0.23	42	0.009	91	41	3.8	1.7	5.0	2.5

bw, body weight; Cn, column; CV, coefficient of variation; DF, degrees of freedom; F, fluoride; h, hour; m, minute; MS, Microsoft; ppm, parts per million; SD, standard deviation; SE, standard error; y, year

Four children were aged 4 years, and two were aged 5 years.
The accurate mean age is 4.3 + 0.5 = 4.8
Example: age 5 at last birthday in fact means and age range from 5.00 to 5.99; therefore, 0.5 years must be added

Formulae
Cn 17 = Cn 14 × Cn 15
Cn 18 = 24/Cn 16
Cn 19 = Cn 14 × Cn 18
Cn 20 = Cn 17 × Cn 18

Confidence limits, p = 0.95
t for p = 0.05, DF = N-1: 2.570

	Cn19	Cn20	Cn21	Cn22	Cn23	Cn24
Lower limit	476	183	19.8	7.6	23.9	8.7
Upper limit	943	396	39.3	16.5	49.4	21.4

Table 7.7 Dataset example and MS Excel computing table showing calculations of fluoride excreti of children providing nocturnal and noon urine collections

Enter source of data and a summary of fluoride exposure here

Enter source of data here (example of 10 subjects for illustration; No. 85 with "easy" data) and case 91 zero valid collections

Personal data					Night										
Subject ID No.	Sex M = 1 F = 2	Age (yrs)	Bw (kg)	Subject No.	Field and laboratory data				Valid "=1"	Valid time at initial void Ing(hhmm)	Duration of collection hh.dec	Results per			
					Time at initial voiding (hhmm)	Collection ended (hhmm)	Urine volume (mL)	F conc (ppm)				Urine flow (mL/h)	F excr. (µg/h)	Sub No.
Cn1	Cn2	Cn3	Cn4	Cn11	Cn12	Cn13	Cn14	Cn15	Cn16	Cn17	Cn18	Cn19	Cn20	Cn2
81	1	3.7	15	81	1830	720	300	1.06	1	1830	12.83	23.4	24.8	81
82	1	3.4		82	1600	705	150	1.59	1	1600	15.08	9.9	15.8	82
83	1	5	17	83	2400	930	220	0.533	1	2400	9.50	23.2	12.3	83
84	1	4	16	84			200	1.29	0	x	x	x	x	84
85	1	3.3	16	85	2040	640	240	0.5	1	2040	10.00	24.0	12.0	85
87	1	5	18	87			320	1.85	0	x	x	x	x	87
88	2	3.6	16	88	2040	700	300	0.53	1	2040	10.33	29.0	15.4	88
91	1	5	20	91	2000				0	x	x	x	x	91
89	1	3.6	17	89	1910	715	200	1.1	1	1910	12.08	16.6	18.2	89
90	2	3.8	15	90	1400	2100	300	0.766	1	1400	7.00	42.9	32.8	90
10	N	10	9	N	8	7	9	9	7	7	7	7	7	N
Min		3	15	Min	1400	640	150.0	0.500		1400	7.0	9.9	12.0	Min
Max		5	20	Max	2400	2100	320.0	1.85		2400	15.1	42.9	32.8	Max
Median		4	16	Median	1955	715	240.0	1.060		1910	10.3	23.4	15.8	Med
Mean		4.0	16.6	Mean			247.8	1.024			11.0	24.1	18.8	Mea
	SD	0.7	1.6	SD				0.488			2.6	10.3	7.5	SD
If age only in integers:				CV				48			24	43	40	CV
Raw mean age														
Plus 0.5:		4.5		CV = 100 × SD/Mean										

Time of voiding the bladder: between 0001 and 2400 (0000 will invalidate the case)

bw, body weight; Cn, column; CV, coefficient of variation; DF, degrees of freedom; F, fluoride; h, hour; ID, identification; m, minute; MS, Microsoft; ppm, parts per mil SD, standard deviation; SE, standard error; y, year

Gender of subjects			Row 10 provides column numbers	Explanation formulae	Total number of subjects
	N	%	Leave blank those cells of the field	Cn 18 = duration of collection in hours and decimals	Subjects with at least 1 valid collection
Female	2	20	and laboratory data where the data	Cn 19 = Cn14/Cn18	Number of subject with all collections valid
Male	8	80	is missing. Collections are only	Cn 20 = Cn 14 × Cn 15/Cn18	Number of valid collections
Sum	10	100	valid where all four sets of field and laboratory data are recorded		Number of collections per subject, mean

	Field and laboratory data			Valid "=1"	Valid time at initial voiding (hhmm)	Duration of collection (hh.dec)	Results per h			No. of valid collections (Cn16 + Cn 26)
...me at ...ial ...ding mm)	Collection ended (hhmm)	Urine volume (mL)	F conc. (ppm)				Urine flow (mL/h)	F excr. (µg/h)	No	
22	Cn23	Cn24	Cn25	Cn26	Cn27	Cn28	Cn29	Cn30	Cn31	Cn32
0	1530	70	0.922	1	1200	3.50	20.0	18.4	**81**	2
0	1440	140	1.42	1	1200	2.67	52.5	74.6	**82**	2
5	1500	100	1.18	1	1145	3.25	30.8	36.3	**83**	2
0	1520	170	1.41	1	1200	3.33	51.0	71.9	**84**	1
0	1500	90	2	1	1200	3.00	30.0	60.0	**85**	2
0	1530	70	1.25	1	1220	3.17	22.1	27.6	**87**	1
0	1450	170	0.843	1	1200	2.83	60.0	50.6	**88**	2
0	1400			0	x	x	x	x	**91**	0
0	1330	90	1.45	1	1210	1.33	67.5	97.9	**89**	2
0	1320	220	1.2	1	1200	1.33	165.0	198.0	**90**	2
0	**10**	**9**	**9**	**9**	**9**	**9**	**9**	**9**		**16**
5	1320	70.0	0.843		1145	1.3	20.0	18.4		
0	1530	220.0	2.000		1220	3.5	165.0	198.0		
0	1475	100.0	1.250		1200	3.0	51.0	60.0		
		124.4	**1.297**			**2.7**	**55.4**	**70.6**		
			0.339			0.8	44.5	53.9		
			26			3.0	80	76		

Table 7.8 Dataset example and MS Excel computing table showing calculations of fluoride excreti(on) of children providing morning, afternoon and nocturnal collections

Enter source of data and a summary of fluoride exposure here

Enter source of data here — (Ten subjects for illustration: case 59 with "easy" data)

Subject No. (cn1)	Gender m=1 f=2 (cn2)	Age, yrs (cn3)	Body weight kg (cn4)	Coded individual fluoride exposure	No. (cn11)	Time at initial voiding hhmm (cn12)	Collection ended hhmm (cn13)	Urine volume ml (cn14)	F conc. ppm (cn15)	Valid "=1" (cn16)	Valid time at initial voiding hhmm (cn17)	Duration of collection hh.dec (cn18)	Urine flow ml/h (cn19)	F excr. µg/h (cn20)	No. (cn21)	Time at initial voiding hhmm (cn22)	Collection ended hhm (cn23)
								MORNING		Valid "=1"			*MORNING*			*AFTERNOO(N)*	
53	2	4	25		53	900	1114	240	0.16	1	900	2.23	107.5	17.1	53	1330	145
54	1	5			54	907	1107	35	0.34	1	907	2.00	17.5	5.9	54	1334	150
56	2	5	27		56	900	1100	60	0.5	1	900	2.00	30.0	15.0	56	1320	152
57	1	4	19		57	855		17	0.46	0	x	x	x	x	57	1330	151
58	1	4	22		58	900	1116	75	0.34	1	900	2.27	33.1	11.3	58	1335	150
59		4	20		59	1000	1100	100	0.2	1	1000	1.00	100.0	20.0	59	1330	153
60	1	5	17		60					0	x	x	x	x	60	1334	150
61	2	5	23		61	911	1118	10	0.31	1	911	2.12	4.7	1.4	61	1335	150
62	1	4	23		62	914	1110	40	0.97	1	914	1.93	20.7	20.1	62	1350	
63	2	4	20		63	925	1100	60	0.72	1	925	1.58	37.9	27.3	63	1355	151
10	N	10	9		N	9	8	9	9	8	8	8	8	8	10	9	
	Min	4.0	17.0		Min	855	1100	10.0	0.159		900	1.00	4.7	1.4	Min	1320	1459
	Max	5.0	27.0		Max	1000	1118	240.0	0.970		1000	2.27	107.5	27.3	Max	1355	1530
	Median	4.0	22.0		Median	907	1109	60.0	0.340		909	2.00	31.5	16.0	Med.	1334	1504
	Mean	4.4	21.8		Mean			70.8	0.443			1.89	43.9	14.8	Mean		
	SD	0.5	3.1		Standard deviation, SD				0.259			0.42	38.4	8.3	SD		
Raw mean age					Coeff. of variation, CV				59			22	87	56	CV		
plus 0.5:		4.9			Standard error, SE				0.086			0.15	13.56	2.95	SE		
					CV = 100*SD/Mean												

Time of voiding the bladder: between 0001 and 2400 (0000 will invalidate the case)

	N	%
Females	3	30
Males	7	70
Sum	10	100

Row 10: cn means column number

Leave blank those cells of the field and laboratory data where the data is missing

Only those collections are valid where all 4 field and laboratory data are recorded

Explanations, formulas

cn18 = duration of collection in hours and decimals

cn19 = cn14/cn18

cn20 = cn14*cn15/cn18

rine lume	F conc. ppm	Valid "=1"	AFTERNOON Valid time at initial voiding hhmm	Duration of collection hh.dec	Values per hour Urine flow ml/h	F excr. µg/h	No.	NIGHT Time at initial voiding hhmm	Collection ended hhmm	Urine volume ml	F conc. ppm	Valid "=1"	NIGHT Valid time at initial voiding hhmm	Duration of collection hh.dec	Values per hour Urine flow ml/h	F excr. µg/h	No.	N of valid collections cn16 plus cn26 plus cn36
24	cn25	cn26	cn27	cn28	cn29	cn30	cn31	cn32	cn33	cn34	cn35	cn36	cn37	cn38	cn39	cn40	cn41	cn42
	0.103	1	1330	1.48	53.9	5.6	53	2210	720	140	0.72	1	2210	9.17	15.3	11.0	53	3
	0.77	1	1334	1.50	63.3	48.8	54	2140	845	170	0.61	1	2140	11.08	15.3	9.4	54	3
0	1.0	1	1320	2.00	50.0	50.0	56	2100	700	200	0.4	1	2100	10.00	20.0	8.0	56	3
	0.74	1	1330	1.67	18.0	13.3	57	2005	750	280	0.41	1	2005	11.75	23.8	9.8	57	2
	1.14	1	1335	1.47	19.1	21.8	58	1735	805	255	0.68	1	1735	14.50	17.6	12.0	58	3
0	0.4	1	1330	2.00	60.0	24.0	59	2100	700	500	0.2	1	2100	10.00	50.0	10.0	59	3
	0.249	1	1334	1.50	63.3	15.8	60	2100	845	170	0.612	1	2100	11.75	14.5	8.9	60	2
	0.36	1	1335	1.47	30.7	11.0	61		820	130	0.72	0	x	x	x	x	61	2
	0.89	0	x	x	x	x	62	2030	830	205	0.76	1	2030	12.00	17.1	13.0	62	2
0	0.255	1	1355	1.33	75.0	19.1	63	2010	830	180	1.31	1	2010	12.33	14.6	19.1	63	3
	10	9	9	9	9	9		9	10	10	10	9	9	9	9	9		26
,0	0.103		1320	1.33	18.0	5.6	Min	1735	700	130.0	0.200		1735	9.17	14.5	8.0		
0.0	1.140		1355	2.00	75.0	50.0	Max	2210	845	500.0	1.310		2210	14.50	50.0	19.1		
,0	0.570		1334	1.50	53.9	19.1	Med	2100	812.5	190.0	0.646		2100	11.75	17.1	10.0		
,2	0.591			1.60	48.2	23.3	Mean			223.0	0.642			11.40	20.9	11.2		
	0.361			0.24	20.7	15.8	SD				0.295			1.58	11.3	3.3		
	61			15	43	68	CV				46			14	54	30		
	0.114			0.08	6.89	5.27	SE				0.093			0.53	3.77	1.11		
													Total number of children:	10				
													Number of valid collections:	26				
													Collections per child:	2.60				

Table 7.9 Ideal format of a dataset to be transferred to an evaluation centre

For designation of columns and data to be entered see **Table 7.6**   The figures (*italics*) in the frames are the dates needed for complete evaluation
F exposure should be entered In columns 5–10 (not shown)
(This line is also reserved for the summary of fluoride exposure (e.g. water; salt; milk; toothpaste and fluoride rinses)

	Subject					Morning — Field and laboratory data					Afternoon — Field and laboratory data					Nocturnal — Field and laboratory data			
ID No.[a]	Sex M=1 F=2	Age (yrs)	Bw (kg)	F expos. No.		ID No.	Time initial voiding (hhmm)	Collect. ended (hhmm)	Urine volume (mL)	Fluoride concent. ppm	ID No.	Time initial voiding (hhmm)	Collect. ended (hhmm)	Urine volume (mL)	Fluoride concent. (ppm)	ID No.	Time initial voiding (hhmm)	Collect. ended (hhmm)	Urine volume (mL)	Fluoride concent. (ppm)
Cn1	Cn2	Cn3	Cn4	Cn5	Cn11															
23	1	5	22			23	910	1120	24	0.22	23	1320	1510	85	0.1	23	2150	720	160	0.15
24	2	5	24			24	910	1100	60	0.43	24	1320	1520	65	0.77	24	2200	845	122	0.7
25	2	4	19			25	915	1050	70	0.55	25	1330	1515	48	1.0	25	2130	700	180	0.45
27	1	6	28			27	915	1115	25	0.22	27	1310	1518	30	0.74	27	2115	750	170	0.65
28	2	5	23			28	840	1100	75	0.32	28	1310	1520	45	1.14	28	2050	805	240	0.92
29	1	6	20			29	850	1100	60	0.79	29	1300	1500	82	0.25	29	2155	845	220	0.3
31	1	4	19			31	905	1110	48	0.105	31	1335	1506	64	0.36	31		820-	155	0.27
33	2	4	20			33	910	1110	45	0.46	33					33	2045	830	260	0.45
34	2	5	26			34	850	1100	76	0.87	34	1340	1520	100	0.96	34	2135	830	225	1.2
N						9	9	9	9		8	8	8	8		8	9	9	9	
Min							840	1050	24.0	0.105		1300	1500	30.0	0.103		2045	700	122.0	0.150
Max							915	1120	76.0	0.870		1340	1520	100.0	1.140		2200	845	260.0	1.200
Med							910	1105	60.0	0.430		1320	1517	64.5	0.755		2133	820	180.0	0.450
Mean									**53.7**	**0.441**				**64.9**	**0.665**				**192.4**	**0.566**
SD										0.261					0.382					0.337

bw, body weight; Cn, column; F, fluoride; h, hour; ID, identification; m, minute; MS, Microsoft; ppm, parts per million; SD, standard deviation; y, year
a ID No. is mandatory for Cn1, optional for further columns
Leave blank those cells where details are missing. Basically, a urine collection is valid only when all four sets of field and laboratory data are available
Note: data stored in MS Excel should be checked as far as is possible in MS Excel. The statistics N, Min, Max, Median, Mean and SD are useful for checking by the field worker, and for checking of correct transfers at the evaluation

8   Urine spot samples

Twenty-four hour urine collection is the most reliable method for estimating urinary excretion of fluoride. However, when it is not feasible to obtain 24-hour urine or shorter time-controlled collections, spot urine samples may be obtained. A spot urine sample is defined as an un-timed "single-void" urine sample. This method is the *least informative method* for studying fluoride exposure, because the amount of fluoride excreted per day or per hour cannot be calculated from the concentration alone.

Spot samples are relatively easy to obtain, and measurement of fluoride concentration is relatively simple. The method can be used in a number of situations. First, the value obtained can be compared with standards (Table 7.4). Urinary fluoride concentrations of 0.8–1.2 mg/L (i.e. ppm) are regarded as indicating optimal exposure to fluoride. Based on a large number of studies, mostly conducted in connection with fluoridated water, these limits have been found to be independent of age (*19, 45, 47, 51, 52, 58, 59*). Second, if repeated over a period of time, the values can rapidly disclose changes in fluoride exposure. Thus, such data can show whether a fluoride-based intervention (in water, salt or milk) has been successful in reaching the target community, or whether a source of excessive fluoride exposure has been successfully removed. Third, if the fluoride concentration in spot samples – obtained, for example, about 6 months after a baseline collection and after introduction of a fluoride-based programme – is 20% higher than the baseline measurement, it would be reasonable to assume that the intake of fluoride has also increased by about 20%.

If spot samples are collected, it is best to take them at several times within a day. Urine that has accumulated in the bladder over a short period may reflect a short-lived peak level of the fluoride concentration. Hence, the longer the urine is retained in the bladder, the more representative it is of 24-hour results. For each spot sample, the hour when it was obtained should be recorded. When spot samples are collected in a follow-up assessment of urinary fluoride, the time of day at which the urine is passed should be approximately equal to the collection times in the initial excretion study. In programmes where fluoride is given once or twice per day, spot urine samples are not useful unless they are scheduled in such a way as to be directly associated with the fluoride intake.

8.1 Creatinine

In healthy subjects, urinary creatinine excretion is fairly constant throughout the day. Creatinine concentration in urine is measured in most hospitals or laboratories as a routine test for evaluating kidney function, and the test is easy and relatively cheap. Due to the relative stability of creatinine within an individual, it has also been used for normalization of analytic concentrations. An estimate of 24-hour urinary excretion of fluoride can be calculated by multiplying the ratio of urinary fluoride to urinary creatinine (F: Cr ratio) with creatinine reference values. The mean 24-hour urinary creatinine value of 15 mg/kg bw/day (with 5th and 95th percentiles of 8 and 22 mg/kg bw/day) has been reported as the standard urinary excretion of creatinine (*60*). Also, a mean F: Cr ratio of 1.49 mg F/g Cr has been reported for children (*22*). In young children on a customary diet, good agreement has been reported between the measured 24-hour urinary fluoride excretion and the predicted 24-hour urinary fluoride excretion from the F: Cr ratio (*22*).

9   Provision of technical advice

WHO is willing to help in identifying experts who can assist countries in designing, directing or evaluating data from fluoride exposure studies. Contact the WHO Oral Health Programme, Department for Prevention of Non-communicable Diseases:

World Health Organization
20 Avenue Appia
CH-1211 Geneva – Switzerland
oralhealth@who.int

Apparatus and materials

Specific ion electrodes are used to determine fluoride in water and monitor renal fluoride excretion in community prevention programmes. The following apparatus and elements are needed for the procedure.

1) Polypropylene tubes, 15 mL with screw cap for fluoride determination in urine and water.

2) Disposable gloves to fit hand size of the operator.

3) Disposable paper towels.

4) Climate-controlled room. If tests are to be conducted in a laboratory, ambient conditions are usually maintained at 23 ± 2°C and 50 ± 10% relative humidity; this corresponds roughly to "normal room temperature" in moderate climates, and most laboratories aim to maintain such environmental conditions. Fluoride determination can be conducted at the school or preschool site, if a suitable room is available. However, temperature fluctuation during the day can cause erratic readings – for example, a 1°C difference in temperature will give rise to a measurement error of about 2% – therefore, care must be taken to ensure that standard solutions (used for calibrating electrodes) and urine tests samples are at the same temperature. It is also important to note that lower or higher temperature affects the electrode slope; the slope of the fluoride electrode at 25°C should be 59.2 mV.

5) Running water and accessibility to a drain for disposing of urine after tests are conducted.

6) Distilled or deionized water to prepare standards and solutions (about 20 L, depending on the number of test samples to be evaluated). The number of fluoride determinations can be calculated by taking into consideration:
   - the number of participating subjects – children or adults;
   - the number of collection periods included in the study;
   - all cylinders (tubes) of drinking water brought by subjects; and
   - urine collections taken at the school or at the institution or place of employment if participants are adults.

7) Reliable pH/ISE meter compatible for use with specific fluoride ion electrodes, and to determine the pH of urine if required. Models that have been found to be reliable and simple to use include the Orion Model 720A Plus (available either for 220 or 110 volts operation) or the Orion Dual Star pH/ISE meter (Thermo-Orion Scientific, Beverly, MA, USA). The latter model comes with a universal power supply, with an adapter that has plugs to fit a variety of electric sockets; also, the input voltage can be either 110 or 220 volts. The meter sensitivity can be set to record one, two or three decimal points, depending on the precision desired. For calculation of fluoride excretion rates, meter sensitivity can be set to the nearest 0.01 ppm.

8) Reliable specific fluoride ion electrode. For example, the Orion 9609BN (Thermo-Orion Scientific, Beverly, MA, USA) has been found to be a reliable instrument. Two electrodes are recommended, to make it easier to obtain two readings from each sample. Again, the meter sensitivity can be set to record one, two or three decimal, depending on the precision desired. For calculation of fluoride excretion rates, meter sensitivity can be set to the nearest 0.01 ppm.

9) Reference electrode filling solution, depending on the electrode manufacturer recommendations. If using the Orion electrode, the filling solution recommended is Thermo-Orion Cat 900061.

10) Standard at 100 ppm (e.g. Ion plus Orion 940907).

11) Total ionic strength adjusting buffer (TISAB) to provide a constant background ionic strength, de-complex fluoride and adjust solution pH. Two TISAB buffers can be used: TISAB II for low-level measurements (e.g. Orion 94-09-09) or TISAB III concentrated (Orion 94-09-11).

Note: TISAB II and TISAB III can be prepared from laboratory supplies.

Tisab II

TISAB II is used for most measurements, but is particularly useful in measuring solutions that might have low concentrations of fluoride (<0.4 ppm) and in which no fluoride-complexing agents (e.g. aluminum or iron) are present.

To prepare TISAB II: Place about 500 ml of distilled water in a 1 L beaker. Add 57 mL of glacial acetic acid and 58 g of reagent-grade NaCl. Place the beaker in a water bath for cooling. Immerse a calibrated pH electrode into the solution and slowly add 5 M NaOH until the pH is between 5.0 and 5.5. Cool to room temperature. Pour into a 1 L volumetric flask and dilute to the 1 L mark with distilled water (*61*).

Tisab III

Dissolve 300 g sodium citrate. $2H_2O$ (FW = 294.10), 22 g CDTA, and 60 g NaCl in 1 L water (*62*).

NOTE 2: When the study is conducted in communities that can only be accessed via extensive travel, use of TISAB III concentrated is advantageous because smaller quantities can be transported and are likely to be less expensive. TISAB II is supplied in 3.785 L containers (1 gallon), and it needs to be added to the urine sample in a 1:1 ratio (e.g. add 5 mL of TISAB II to 5 mL of urine). TISAB III is supplied in 500 mL bottles and needs to be added to the urine sample in a 0.1:1 ratio (e.g. add 0.5 mL of TISAB III to 5 mL of urine).

12) Magnetic stirrer with variable speed 110 or 220 volts (e.g. Corning P410).
13) Magnetic micro stirring bars, tetrafluorocarbon coated; 1.6 × 7 mm.
14) Stirring bar retriever, tetrafluorocarbon coated.
15) Plastic beakers, 250 mL capacity (e.g. Fisher Cat 02591–28).
16) Dark plastic bottles, 125 mL with screw cap, for storing standard solutions.
17) One precision micro litre adjustable volume pipette 100–1000 µl (e.g. Brinkman Eppendorf 2100Series Fisher catalogue 05–402–90) with pipette tips (e.g. Brinkman Eppendorf Pipette tips 05–403–26, box of 96) for 100–1000 µl micropipette.
18) One precision micro litre adjustable volume pipette 500–5000 µl (e.g. Brinkman Eppendorf 2100 Series Cat. 05–402–91) with pipette tips (e.g. Brinkman Eppendorf Pipette tips 05–403–71, Rack 5 × 24 = 120) for 500–5000 µl micropipette.
19) One precision micro litre adjustable volume pipette 1–10 mL (e.g. Brinkman Eppendorf 2100 Series Cat 05–403–121 with Brinkman Eppendorf Pipette tips 05–403–116; bulk two bags of 100 = 200) for 1–10 mL micropipette.
20) One plastic or metal test-tube rack with 40 orifices of 17 mm diameter (e.g. Fisher Cat No 14–809B).
21) Semi-logarithmic sheets (three cycles × 70 divisions) (e.g. Keuffel & Esser Co. No 465490).
22) Mini wipes, 10.2 cm, for wiping electrodes after rinsing (e.g. Fisher Cat No. 06–665–28).
23) Class B polypropylene (Nalgene) 100 mL volumetric flasks with polypropylene screw caps (e.g. Fisher 02–617–154).
24) Bimetal thermometer, Celcius scale 0–150°C (e.g. Fisher Catalogue No 15–077–30D).

25) Polyethylene or polypropylene bucket for disposing of urine or water (about 15 L capacity).
26) Electrode stand and holder for two electrodes.
27) Plastic funnel.

Annex B
Steps for verifying function of apparatus

Examine all accessories, instrument (meter) and equipment (electrodes), micropipettes, magnetic stirrer and so on for functional effectiveness before they are used in a test. The electrode chamber must be filled with filling solution about 30–35 minutes (and preferably 1 hour) before its intended use, to allow time for electrode stabilization. The solution level should be at least 25 mm above the level of the sample and the reference junction; the chamber should be filled up to the edge of the hole. The reference junction *must* remain submerged to ensure proper flow rate.

B1 Combination fluoride electrode preparation and checking electrode operation

1. Remove the rubber cap covering the electrode tip.
2. Fill the electrode (for example Model 96–0900 or 9609BN) chamber with special filling solution (for example Catalogue No. 900061) and ensure proper flow rate according to the electrode instruction manual.
3. Connect electrode to the meter.
4. Place 10 mL of distilled water and 10 mL of **TISAB II** into a 25 mL tube or cylinder; or 9 mL of distilled water and 1 mL of **TISAB III** into a 25 mL plastic tube or cylinder.
5. Rinse the electrode with distilled water, blot dry and place into the tube, stir thoroughly, wait for a stable reading and record the electrode potential in millivolts.
6. Pipette 1 mL of 100 ppm standard into the tube or cylinder and stir thoroughly. When a stable reading is displayed, record the electrode potential in millivolts.
7. Pipette 10 mL of the same standard (100 ppm) into the same cylinder and stir thoroughly. When a stable reading is displayed record the electrode potential in millivolts.
8. There should be a 54–60 mV difference between the two millivolt readings when the solution temperature is 20–25 °C. If the millivolt potential

is not within this range, refer to the trouble shooting section of the electrode manual.

This procedure measures the electrode slope, which is defined as the change in millivolts observed every 10-fold change in concentration. Obtaining the slope value is the best way to check electrode operation.

Calibration procedure

C1   Preparation of standards

The standards should bracket the expected sample range; serial dilution is the best method for the preparation of the standards. This can be done starting from a fluoride level of 100 mg/L. The following concentrations are recommended as calibration points: 0.1, 0.5, 1.0 and 5.0 mg F/L. An additional calibration standard of 0.05 mg F/L can also be used. The calibrating solutions of the indicated concentrations can be prepared in relatively small quantities (e.g. 50 or 100 mL) so fresh solutions are always used. Calibration standards can be stored in dark plastic bottles provided with screw cap.

If certified calibrating solutions (per example, Orion) are not available, these can be prepared by starting from a 100 ppm F solution. This solution is commercially available (Orion catalogue No. 940907), or can be prepared (e.g. from a compound of sodium fluoride 100% pure or 99% pure). The reactive should be of high purity (preferably 100% pure). Considering that the molecular weight of the sodium fluoride (NaF) is 42 (19 F and 23 Na), the percentage of the fluoride available would be 45.2%. Hence, if the reactive is only 99% pure, the amount of fluoride would be 44.78%. Thus, in a container of 500 grams, only 223.9 grams are fluoride.

How much of the reactive compound of sodium fluoride needs to be weighed to prepare a solution of fluoride of 100 mg/L, given that in 500 g NaF there are 223.9 g F, and 100 mg F are needed? The calculation indicates that 0.223 g NaF is needed. This amount is deposited in a volumetric flask with a capacity of 1 L, and the flask is filled with distilled water to the 1-L mark.

C1.1   Preparation of standard solutions by serial dilution

From 100 ppm solution takes 10 mL and dilute to 100 mL. This will give a standard of 10 ppm.

From 100 ppm solution takes 5 mL and dilute to 100 mL. This will give a standard of 5 ppm.

To prepare solutions with ppm	To a solution of 10 ppm	Add mL of distilled water to
0.05	0.5	100
0.1	1.0	100
0.5	5.0	100
1.0	10.0	100

ppm, parts per million
Note: It is indispensable to use a micropipette

If numerous determinations are to be made, a larger quantity can be prepared maintaining the same proportions.

The desired amount of calibrating solution is deposited in a plastic container. Thus, for example, for 2 mL, a TISAB II solution in equal amounts (i.e. 2 mL) should be added.

NOTE: If a concentrated TISAB III solution has been added to the standards, this solution should be added to the test samples in the correct proportion (i.e. 1/10 of the amount of standard or sample). **Always use the same type of TISAB in the standards and the sample. Use of TISAB II in the standard and TISAB III in the sample, or vice versa, will cause erroneous concentration readings due to the difference in ionic strength and the dilution factor.**

C2 Actual calibration procedure

The desired amount of calibrating solution (e.g. 5 mL) is deposited in a plastic container, such as a polypropylene tube of 50 mL capacity, and a TISAB II solution in equal amounts (i.e. 5 mL) is added. If a concentrated TISAB III solution is used, then 5 mL of standard solution are placed in the plastic tube and 0.5 mL of TISAB III added.

Note
In many laboratories carrying out fluoride analyses in the context of caries-preventive uses of fluoride, details of the procedures, the types of TISAB and other method details vary to some extent. This is evident from scientific publications that describe the analytical methods in detail. Some specialized laboratories take only 1 mL of urine to be mixed with 1 mL of TISAB

II, to arrive at the 2 mL solution in which the fluoride is measured. Using small quantities, however, requires meticulous work by well-trained laboratory personnel. If, for instance, 0.04 mL of a strong fluoride solution (at, for example, 5 ppm F) is not completely blotted away from the electrode due to less than ideal working conditions, the amount of fluoride in that 0.04 mL will increase the measured concentration in the following urine-TISAB mixture by as much as 0.1 ppm, whereas when working with 5 mL + 5 mL, the concentration is raised only by 0.02 ppm. It is general rule that working with 5 mL + 5 mL is five times less sensitive to imprecise handling than working with 1 mL + 1 mL. Exercising care and good practice, it is possible to use 4 mL (2 mL sample + 2 mL TISAB II) or (4 mL sample + 0.4 mL TISAB III). In this case, 15 mL capacity tubes are suitable for use with the Orion 9609BN ion plus combination electrode. If a different model ion electrode that requires separate reference electrode is used, the size of the plastic cylinder should be large enough to accommodate both electrodes.

54. Determine the standard solution temperature using the thermometer [Annex A24)] and record it in the record book.
55. Deposit the desired amount of standard in separate plastic tubes and label each with the corresponding fluoride concentration.
56. Drop a micro stirring bar into each solution.
57. If two electrodes are to be used, each needs to be calibrated; connect the electrodes to the meter receptacles and note the location of each corresponding channel. If a Orion 720A plus or a Orion Dual Star meter is used, two receptacles are provided in the instrument for connecting two electrodes. Place the electrode inside the tube having the lowest concentration standard (i.e. 0.05 ppm or 0.1 ppm) taking care to maintain the solution level slightly below the electrode chamber's orifice.
58. Start the magnetic stirrer and stir the solution in a low setting. The stirrer platform may become warm, and heat transfer to the test samples will affect the accuracy of the calibration curve. Therefore, prevent heat transfer by placing a piece of cork or board as an insulator between the stirrer platform and the bottom of the test tube.
59. Follow manufacturer's instructions for operation of the meter for calibration procedures in the concentration mode. Each electrode to be used in fluoride determination must be calibrated separately. When a stable reading is observed on the display screen, record the reading. Remove the electrode from the plastic tube, rinse it with distilled or deionized water and blot with fine tissue.

60. Proceed with the next concentration standard (i.e. 0.5) repeating the process until readings from all succeeding standard solutions (1.0, 5.0 and 10.0 ppm) are obtained.
61. If using the Orion Dual Star meter, a calibration curve can be displayed. Although modern meters automatically construct a calibration curve in the meter memory, it is important to be able to construct a calibration curve on semi-logarithmic paper. Electrode potentials of standard solutions are measured and plotted on the linear axis (ordinate) against their concentrations on the long axis (abscissa). The registered values for each standard solution are entered onto semi-logarithmic paper. This can be made in the millivolts or the concentration mode. The values of the obtained reading of each solution are connected by a line. If the electrode is working correctly, and standard solutions properly made, the readings should be connected essentially by a straight line. If calibration is satisfactory, proceed with the next step.

C3 Determination of fluoride in urine and water

If the public health facility has a laboratory or if the oral health personnel desire to conduct the determination of fluoride in urine or water, the following procedure is recommended:

1. Ensure that urine test samples are brought to room temperature, and that their temperature and that of the standard are the same.
2. The person responsible for conducting fluoride determination **must** decide, ahead of time, the quantity of urine sample that will be used in the tests. This quantity regulates the amount of TISAB that will be needed. Further, a decision must be made as to whether TISAB II or TISAB III will be used. The same type of TISAB (II or III) must be added to both standard solutions and urine test samples.
3. Depending of the type of TISAB used (TISAB II or TISAB III), use a micropipette to measure either 5 mL (2 mL or 4 mL if using a 15 mL tube) of urine from the plastic tube containing the samples collected from each child in the corresponding collection period.

> Add either 5 or 2 mL of TISAB II or 0.4 mL of TISAB III to the sample and gently mix it.

2. Drop a mini stirring bar into the sample.
3. Start the magnetic stirrer, set at a low speed. Place the plastic tube containing the sample over it and ensure that the electrode is properly held in place in the electrode stand or holder. Follow the procedures

given by the meter manufacturer to obtain direct readings in the concentration mode.

4. When a stable reading is obtained, record it as the concentration of fluoride in the sample with electrode No. 1.

5. Carefully remove the electrode from the tube containing the sample, rinse the electrode with distilled or deionized water, and blot the electrode, taking care not to rub the lanthanum membrane at the tip of the electrode.

6. Place electrode No. 2, which has been connected to the other channel, and repeat steps 3–5.

The average of the two determinations is recorded as the concentration of fluoride in the urine obtained from the child in the corresponding collection period.

7. Repeat the procedure in an identical manner for each of the urine test samples collected in a given collection period, ensuring that calibration of each electrode is verified every 1.5 hours, or even more frequently if there is any temperature change in the room where tests are being conducted.

The described procedure is identical for determining fluoride concentration in water.

Keep in mind the importance of ensuring that standards and test samples are at the same temperature during measurements (25°C is recommended), and retain a constant stirring speed. Two parallel determinations are made and the average value is calculated and used for further processing.

It is also important to verify the calibration of the electrode every 1.5 hours, or even more frequently if there is any temperature change in the room where tests are being conducted.

NOTE Electrodes do not last indefinitely. Those in regular daily use may often function satisfactorily for 1–2 years, whereas those used intermittently last longer. Indications of breakdown include erratic read-outs taking several minutes to stabilize, and slope out of range (normally 54–50 mV per 10-fold change in F concentration). If such irregularities are observed, electrode replacement is recommended.

References

1 Petersen P.E. *The world oral health report*. WHO/NMH/NPH/ORH/03.2 2003 (http://www.who.int/oral_health/media/en/orh_report03_en.pdf, accessed 10 December 2013).

2 Petersen P.E., Lennon M.A. Effective use of fluorides for the prevention of dental caries in the 21st century: The WHO approach. *Community Dent Oral Epidemiol*, 2004, 32:319–321 (http://www.who.int/entity/oral_health/media/en/orh_cdoe_319to321.pdf, accessed 10 December 2013).

3 *Fluorides and oral health*. Technical Report Series No. 846, Geneva, World Health Organization, 1994 (http://whqlibdoc.who.int/trs/WHO_TRS_846.pdf, accessed 10 December 2013).

4 *Fluoridation and dental health*. WHA28.64, Geneva, World Health Organization, World Health Assembly (WHA), 1975 (http://apps.who.int/iris/bitstream/10665/95721/1/WHA28.64_fre.pdf, accessed 10 December 2013).

5 *Fluoridation and dental health*. WHA22.30, Geneva, World Health Organization, World Health Assembly (WHA), 1969 (http://apps.who.int/iris/bitstream/10665/91255/1/WHA22.30_eng.pdf, accessed 10 December 2013).

6 *Fluorides and the prevention of dental caries*. WHA31.50, Geneva, World Health Organization, World Health Assembly (WHA), 1978 (http://whqlibdoc.who.int/wholis/3/WHA31_R50_eng.pdf, accessed 10 December 2013).

7 *Report on global oral health EB120/10 and draft resolution EB120.R5*. Executive Board Meeting January 2007, Geneva, World Health Organization, 2007 (http://apps.who.int/gb/ebwha/pdf_files/EB120/b120_r5-en.pdf, accessed 10 December 2013).

8 *Oral health: Action plan for promotion and integrated disease prevention*. WHA60.17, Geneva, World Health Organization, World Health Assembly (WHA), 2007 (http://www.healthsystemsevidence.org/R.aspx?U=-1&T=EXTERNAL&A=21036&D=FreeFullText-Full-text+report+(free)&L=http%3a%2f%2fapps.who.int%2fgb%2febwha%2fpdf_files%2fWHASSA_WHA60-Rec1%2fE%2fWHASS1_WHA60REC1-en.pdf, accessed 10 December 2013).

9 Marthaler T.M., Petersen P.E. Salt fluoridation – an alternative in automatic prevention of dental caries. *Int Dent J*, 2005, 55(6):351–358 (http://www.who.int/oral_health/publications/orh_IDJ_salt_fluoration.pdf, accessed 10 December 2013).

10 *Milk fluoridation for the prevention of dental caries.* In: Bánóczy J, Petersen PE & Rugg-Gunn AJ, eds. Geneva, World Health Organization, 2009 (http://www.who. int/oral_health/publications/milk_fluoridation_2009_en.pdf, accessed 10 December 2013).

11 Marthaler T.M. *Monitoring of renal fluoride excretion in community prevention programes on oral health.* WHO/NCD/NCS/ORH/99-1, Geneva, World Health Organization, 1999.

12 *Oral health surveys: Basic methods* (5ᵗʰ Edition). Geneva, World Health Organization, 2013 (http://apps.who.int/iris/handle/10665/41905, accessed 13 December 2013).

13 Murray J.J. *Appropriate use of fluorides for human health.* Geneva, World Health Organization, 1986 (http://whqlibdoc.who.int/publications/1986/9241542039_ (part1).pdf, accessed 10 December 2013).

14 Rugg-Gunn A.J., Villa A.E., Buzalaf M.R. Contemporary biological markers of exposure to fluoride. *Monogr Oral Sci*, 2011, 22:37–51.

15 Buzalaf M.A.R., Rodrigues M., Pessan J., Leite A., Arana A., Villena R. et al. Biomarkers of fluoride in children exposed to different sources of fluoride. *J Dent Res*, 2011, 90(2):215–219.

16 Pessan J.P., Buzalaf M.R. Historical and recent biological markers of exposure to fluoride. *Monogr Oral Sci*, 2011, 22:52–65.

17 Villa A., Anabalon M., Zohouri V., Maguire A., Franco A.M., Rugg-Gunn A. Relationships between fluoride intake, urinary fluoride excretion and fluoride retention in children and adults: An analysis of available data. *Caries Res*, 2010, 44(1):60–68

18 Levy S.M., Kiritsy M.C., Warren J.J. Sources of fluoride intake in children. *J Public Health Dent*, 1995, 55(1):39–52.

19 Rugg-Gunn A.J., Nunn J.H., Ekanayake L., Saparamadu K.D., Wright W.G. Urinary fluoride excretion in 4-year-old children in Sri Lanka and England. *Caries Res*, 1993, 27(6):478–483.

20 Baez R.J., Podairu A., Marthaler T.M., Baez M.X., Floarea L. Urinary fluoride excretion by children and elderly individuals in Romania (Timisoara and Bucharest). *Oral Health and Dental Management in the Black Sea Countries*, 2007, 6(3[21]):3–11 (http://www.oralhealth.ro/volumes/2007/volume-3/V3-07-1.pdf, accessed 10 December 2013).

21 Zohouri F.V., Rugg-Gunn A.J. Total fluoride intake and urinary excretion in 4-year-old Iranian children residing in low-fluoride areas. *Br J Nutr*, 2000, 83(1):15–25.

22 Zohouri F.V., Swinbank C.M., Maguire A., Moynihan P.J. Is the fluoride/creatinine ratio of a spot urine sample indicative of 24-h urinary fluoride? *Community Dent Oral Epidemiol*, 2006, 34(2):130–138.

23 Ketley C.E., Cochran J.A., Lennon M.A., O'Mullane D.M., Worthington H.V. Urinary fluoride excretion of young children exposed to different fluoride regimes. *Community Dental Health*, 2002, 19(1):12–17.

24 Acevedo A.M., Febres-Cordero C., Feldman S., Arasme M.A., Pedauga D.F., Gonzalez H. et al. Urinary fluoride excretion in children aged 3 to 5 years exposed to fluoridated salt at 60 to 90 mgF/Kg in two Venezuelan cities. A pilot study. *Acta Odontol Latinoam*, 2007, 20(1):9–16.

25 Ketley C.E., Cochran J.A., Holbrook W.P., Sanches L., van Loveren C., Oila A.M. et al. Urinary fluoride excretion by preschool children in six European countries. *Community Dent Oral Epidemiol*, 2004, 32:62–68.

26 Franco A.M., Martignon S., Saldarriaga A., Gonzalez M.C., Arbelaez M.I., Ocampo A. et al. Total fluoride intake in children aged 22–35 months in four Colombian cities. *Community Dent Oral Epidemiol*, 2005, 33(1):1–8.

27 Haftenberger M., Viergutz G., Neumeister V., Hetzer G. Total fluoride intake and urinary excretion in German children aged 3–6 years. *Caries Res*, 2001, 35(6): 451–457.

28 Villa A., Anabalon M., Cabezas L. The fractional urinary fluoride excretion in young children under stable fluoride intake conditions. *Community Dent Oral Epidemiol*, 2000, 28(5):344–355.

29 Ekstrand J., Fomon S.J., Ziegler E.E., Nelson S.E. Fluoride pharmacokinetics in infancy. *Pediatric Research*, 1994, 35(2):157–163.

30 Maguire A., Zohouri F.V., Hindmarch P.N., Hatts J., Moynihan P.J. Fluoride intake and urinary excretion in 6- to 7-year-old children living in optimally, sub-optimally and non-fluoridated areas. *Community Dent Oral Epidemiol*, 2007, 35(6):479–488.

31 Grijalva-Haro M.I., Barba-Leyva M.E., Laborin-Alvarez A. Fluoride intake and excretion in children of Hermosillo, Sonora, Mexico. *Salud Publica de Mexico*, 2001, 43(2):127–134.

32 Ekstrand J., Hardell L.I., Spak C.J. Fluoride balance studies on infants in a 1-ppm-water-fluoride area. *Caries Res*, 1984, 18(1):87–92.

33 Villa A.E., Salazar G., Anabalon M., Cabezas L. Estimation of the fraction of an ingested dose of fluoride excreted through urine in pre-school children. *Community Dent Oral Epidemiol*, 1999, 27(4):305–312.

34 Ketley C.E., Lennon M.A. Determination of fluoride intake from urinary fluoride excretion data in children drinking fluoridated school milk. *Caries Res*, 2001, 35(4):252–257.

35 Pessan J.P., Pin M.L.G., Martinhon C.C.R., de Silva S.M.B., Granjeiro J.M., Buzalaf M.A. Analysis of fingernails and urine as biomarkers of fluoride exposure from dentifrice and varnish in 4- to 7-year-old children. *Caries Res*, 2005, 39(5): 363–370.

36 Villa A., Anabalon M., Cabezas L., Rugg-Gunn A. Fractional urinary fluoride excretion of young female adults during the diurnal and nocturnal periods. *Caries Res*, 2008, 42(4):275–281.

37 Villa A., Cabezas L., Anabalon M., Garza E. The fractional urinary fluoride excretion of adolescents and adults under customary fluoride intake conditions, in a

community with 0.6-mg F/L in its drinking water. *Community Dental Health*, 2004, 21(1):11–18.

38   Spencer H., Lewin I., Wistrowski E., Samachson J. Fluoride metabolism in man. *Am J Med*, 1970, 49(6):807–813.

39   Maheshwari U.R., King J., Brunetti A.J., Hodge H.C., Newbrun E., Margen S. Fluoride balances in pregnant and nonpregnant women. *J Occup Med*, 1981, 23(7):465–468 (http://www.ncbi.nlm.nih.gov/pubmed/?term=Fluoride+balances+ in+pregnant+and+nonpregnant+women, accessed 13 December 2013).

40   Spencer H., Kramer L., Osis D., Wiatrowski E. Excretion of retained fluoride in man. *J App Physiol*, 1975, 38(2):282–287.

41   Bingham S., Cummings J.H. The use of 4-aminobenzoic acid as a marker to validate the completeness of 24 h urine collections in man. *Clin Sci*, 1983, 64(6):629–635.

42   Jakobsen J., Ovesen L., Fagt S., Pedersen A.N. Para-aminobenzoic acid used as a marker for completeness of 24 hour urine: assessment of control limits for a specific HPLC method. *Eur J Clin Nutr*, 1997, 51(8):514–519.

43   Baez R.J., Marthaler T.M., Baez M.X., Warpeha R.A. Urinary fluoride levels in Jamaican children after 21 years of salt fluoridation. *Schweiz Monatsschr Zahnmed*, 2010, 120:21–28.

44   Marthaler T.M. Urinary fluoride in pre-school children related to use of fluoridated milk or salt. *Caries Res*, 1994, 28:217.

45   Marthaler T.M., Binder-Fuchs M., Baez R.J., Menghini G. Urinary fluoride excretion in Swiss children aged 3 and 4 consuming fluoridated domestic salt. 2000, 5:9–17.

46   Marthaler T.M., Steiner M., Menghini G., De Crousaz P. Urinary fluoride excretion in children with low fluoride intake or consuming fluoridated salt. *Caries Res*, 1995, 29(1):26–34.

47   Baez R.J., Baez M.X., Marthaler T.M. Urinary fluoride excretion by children 4–6 years old in a south Texas community. 2000, 7(4):242–248.

48   Phantumvanit P., Sangkheaw S., Lekfuengfu P., Niyomsilp K. Urinary fluoride excretion in children drinking fluoridated school milk in Thailand. *Oral Health and Dental Management in the Black Sea Countries*, 2007, 6(2):12–20.

49   Steiner M. Fluoridausscheidung im Urin von Schulkindern im Zusammenhang mit der Speisesalzfuoridierung (Urinary fluoride excretion in children in relation to salt fluoridation). 1985, 95:1109–1117.

50   Marthaler T.M., Menghinin G.D., Steiner M., Sener-Zanola B., De Crousaz P. Excrecion urinaria de fluoruro en ninos suizos que consumen suplementos de fluoruro en la sal o el agua (Urinary fluoride excretions in Swiss children consuming supplemental fluoride in salt or drinking water). 1992, 4:27–35.

51   Pucci F.W., Dol I. *Estudio de excrecion urinaria de fluor en niños de 3 a 5 anos (A study of urinary fluoride excretion in children aged 3 to 5 years)*. Uruguay, Ministerio de Salud Publica (Ministry of Public Health), 1997.

52 Szekely M., Banoczy J., Fazakas Z., Hobai S., Villa A. A comparison of two methods for the evaluation of the daily urinary fluoride excretion in Romanian pre-school children. *Community Dental Health*, 2008, 25(1):23–27.

53 Hetzer G., Straube H., Neumeister V. Zur Verwendung fluoridierten Speisesalzes in der Gemeinschaftsvepflegung (About the use of fluoridated salt in canteens). *Dtsch Zahnarztl Z*, 1996, 51:679–682.

54 *Sodium intake in populations: Assessment of evidence.* Institute of Medicine of the National Academies, 1988 (http://www.iom.edu/~/media/Files/Report%20Files/2013/Sodium-Intake-Populations/SodiumIntakeinPopulations_RB.pdf, accessed 13 December 2013).

55 Smith S.M., Nillen J.L. *Urine preservative: Patent 6261844.* July 17 2001 (http://www.patentstorm.us/patents/6261844/description.html, accessed 10 December 2013).

56 Neefus J.D., Cholak J., Saltzman B.E. The determination of fluoride in urine using a fluoride-specific ion electrode. *Am Ind Hyg Assoc J*, 1970, 31(1):96–99.

57 Obry-Musset A.M., Bettembourg D., Cahen P.M., Voegel J.C., Frank R.M. Urinary fluoride excretion in children using potassium fluoride containing salt or sodium fluoride supplements. *Caries Res*, 1992, 26(5):367–370.

58 Zohouri F.V. *Fluoride intake and excretion in 4-year-old Iranian children.* PhD thesis, United Kingdom, University of Newcastle, 1997.

59 Rugg-Gunn A.J., Al-Mohammadi S.M., Butler T.J. Malnutrition and developmental defects of enamel in 2- to 6-year-old Saudi boys. *Caries Res*, 1998, 32(3): 181–192.

60 Tietz N.W. *Clinical guide to laboratory tests.* Philadelphia, W.B. Saunders, 1983.

61 Orion Research. Analysis methods by pH and ion selective electrodes. Beverly, Massachusetts, 2011 (http://delloyd.50megs.com/moreinfo/ISE.html, accessed January 2012).

62 Analytical Chemistry Resources. Analysis methods by pH and ion selective electrodes. Delloyd's Lab Tech resources reagents and solutions (http://delloyd.50megs.com/moreinfo/ISE.html, accessed).